The New

Fertility Diet Guide

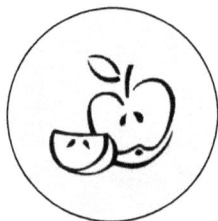

Delicious
FOOD SECRETS
That Can Help You Get Pregnant Faster
At Any Age!

Getting Pregnant:

The New

𝓕ertility 𝓓iet 𝓖uide

By Niels H. Lauersen, M.D.,Ph.D
& Colette Bouchez

Ivy League Press
New York, NY

ILP

The New Fertility Diet Guide

Copyright 2009 Niels H. Lauersen & Colette Bouchez

The New Fertility Diet Guide may be purchased for business or promotional use or special sales. For information please contact Info@IvyLeaguePress.com or visit www.IvyLeaguePress.com

This book is not intended as a substituted for medical advice from your physician. The reader should regularly consult with a physician in matters relating to her health and fertility, particularly in respect to symptoms that
may require medical attention.

The authors, or Ivy League Press cannot be responsible for any results obtained or derived from information in this book.
The information in this book is not considered medical advice and is offered only as a nutritional guide.

Printed in the United States of America 10
9 8 7 6 5 4 3 2 1
First Edition Published 2009

ISBN: 978-0615323237

Library of Congress Cataloging in Publication Data :
The New Fertility Guide/Niels Lauersen - Colette Bouchez
1. Conception - Popular works 2. Reproductive Health- Popular works - 3. Diet and Nutrition - Popular Works

Interior & Cover Design by www. ElleMedia.info

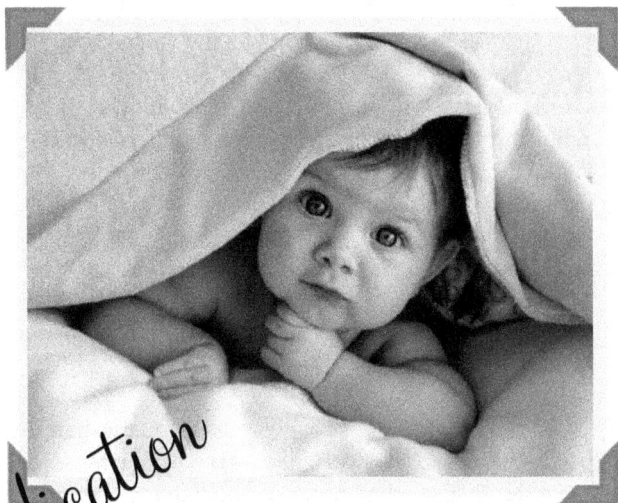

Dedication

This book is dedicated to all the beautiful new babies born this year and to their brand new moms, who believed in the power of diet to help them get pregnant.

And... to all the beautiful new babies - and the the smart & healthy new moms to come!

Acknowledgements

First and foremost we would like to thank all the thousands of patients who, throughout the years, helped us test and perfect our fertility diet. Your wonderful pregnancy success stories have been our inspiration and we can't thank you enough.

To the many medical and health organizations who saw the need to go forward with dedicated research on the power of nutrition, and especially to those who recognized the important links between diet and fertility, we offer our most sincere thanks.

We are also indebted to all those who so generously shared with us their expertise, but most especially The American Society of Reproductive Medicine, the American Dietetic Association, The American Diabetes Association, The Society for Food Information and Technology and The American College of Obstetricians and Gynecologists.

To all our colleagues in the brave new world-wide community of fertility medicine, thank you for helping us carry our message of nutritional hope and help to so many of your patients. We are grateful for your support and encouragement.

And finally, to the staff of Ivy League Press: We are grateful for all your support, dedication and hard work to bring this book to fruition. It was truly a labor of love. And to St. Jude: Thank you for watching over us and keeping us strong.

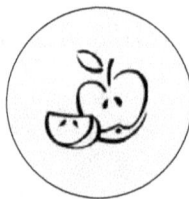

The New

Fertility Diet Guide

By Niels H. Lauersen, MD, PhD & Colette Bouchez

Table Of Contents

INTRODUCTION:

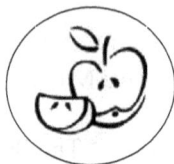

Feed Your Fertility: The Secret To Getting Pregnant Fast!

Getting pregnant, and building a family is one of the most beautiful ways that two partners can express their love for each other - and bring unbounded joy into their lives!

And while we often don't look at it quite this way, having a baby is really what "boy meets girl" is all about! It's why we are attracted to our mate to begin with, and it's how and why that attraction stirs not only our emotions but also our physical desires.

In fact, some of that special magic that drew you and your life partner together is also a part of the chemistry that will eventually draw his sperm to your egg. And when they meet - well that's when the real magic happens: A baby is created!

Now imagine if there was a way to make that fertility magic happen even quicker and easier ...and help ensure that all your sweet baby dreams come true even sooner than you thought?

Well I am here to tell you that there is a way – and it's as close as your dinner plate!

I'm talking about the enormous role we now now that food - and specifically certain foods - can play in not only increasing your fertility, but in helping you get pregnant faster and easier. In fact research now shows that some of these foods may even help ensure you give birth to a healthier and smarter baby!

And when you think about it, the very idea that food can impact fertility is right in line with what we're been discovering about the powerful role that nutrition can play in helping us overcome and even prevent many health threats. We now know for example, that there are clear and direct connections between the foods that we eat and the prevention and even the treatment of heart disease, high blood pressure, diabetes and even some types of cancer.

The very latest research shows that there may even be links between diet and auto-immune diseases most likely to impact women, such as multiple sclerosis, lupus and fibromyalgia.

Having grown up and received my medical training in Denmark

Making just a few changes in your diet can have a powerful effect on your ability to get pregnant quicker & easier!

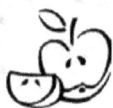

> *More and more evidence is coming to light proving that what you eat can impact your fertility & make a difference in how quickly you get pregnant.*

and other European countries –where diet has long   played a key role in health care - I can't say I am completely surprised by the new findings. But I can say that I am excited and proud beyond belief that so many of these new studies back and support   the very same *nutritional secrets* that I have used to help thousands of my patients get pregnant faster and easier – even those patients who were older, or whose reproductive status was less than optimal.

Indeed, throughout the years my patients continued to prove over and over that not only can diet play a key role in getting pregnant, but more importantly , key nutrients found in certain foods can help overcome even difficult fertility odds.

Equally important is the concept of "food synergy". This is the science of how foods work together to achieve specific results. Although it's now one of the hottest trends in nutrition, I discovered long ago the power of "food synergy" to multiply many times over the power of individual nutrients to enhance fertility.

And in this book I will not only teach you about food synergy, but also fill you in on all the powerful fertility food secrets that I have seen - and research has shown - can make a huge difference in your ability to get pregnant.

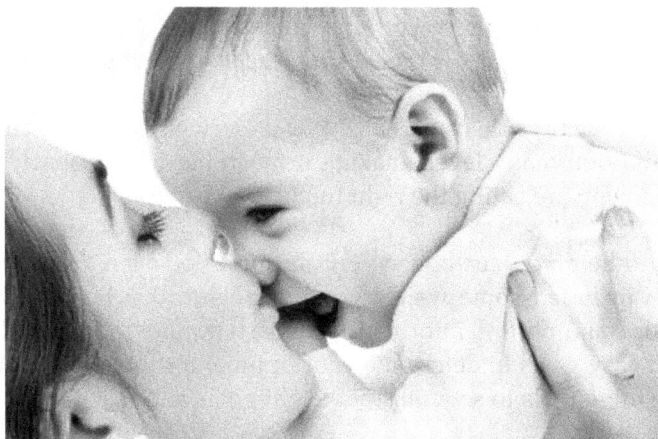

Your Fertility Diet - Your Way!

One of the things my patients have always loved about my fertility food plan is not only that is it is so easy to follow, but that it offers the freedom and the flexibility to choose the foods you love and to eat them at any meal you like!

In fact, if you follow the guidelines in this book you will soon be able to write your own " Fertility Prescription" and create fertility-boosting meal plans based on the foods you love.

Indeed, by showing you how easy it can be to create meals based on a variety of food groups that work together to encourage fertility, you will have both the information and the tools to customize your own fertility diet plan - one that is based on the foods you and your partner love the most!

To help you succeed even faster and easier, at the end of this book you will also find lists of individual "fertility foods" along with nutritional tips related to every food group mentioned in the book, which can make planning your "fertility meals" even easier.

Moreover, as some of you may already know, weight can play a significant role in how quickly and easily you get pregnant.

In fact, being either overweight or underweight can interfere with fertility on many levels making it much harder to conceive - even when you are eating the right foods.

So, to help you customize your fertility food plan even more, I've also included some weight control tools in this book - including calorie and portion information for each fertility food as well as fast and easy ways to determine your optimal fertility weight. You can use these tools to set your set weight goals and reach them quickly and easily.

But in addition to all this information I've also included something else that I hope you will find helpful - a chapter on some of the newest information about how conception occurs, and more importantly, what can stand in the way. I believe that having this information will help you to better understand all the ways that diet and lifestyle changes can influence your fertility - and how important even small changes can be.

Ultimately I am quite certain that regardless of your fertility status right now, this information, together with all the nutritional secrets you will find in this book, will not only help you get pregnant faster, but also improve your overall health in the process.

Of course like all important changes in your life, most of the really big differences in your health or your fertility won't occur overnight. While I do believe you will begin to feel better in just a week or two of making these dietary changes it's important to realize that it could take one or two cycles before you see a measurable difference in your ability to conceive.

That said, if you are willing to put in the time and the small bit of effort to make these changes, I can promise you that *change will come* - not only to your fertility, but also your overall health! And perhaps most importantly, you will forever see those changes reflected in the smile of your brand beautiful new baby!

CHAPTER ONE:

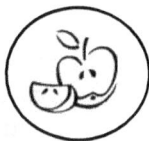

Getting Pregnant: What You Need To Know

While the creation of the universe has been a long standing topic of great debate, I've always believed that the ultimate answer lies within a woman's body. Because it is here that you will find find the very essence of how all life begins. I'm talking about the "egg." Developed, nurtured and "hatched" inside your ovary, each tiny but miraculous egg contains the basis of all life, including one-half of all the DNA necessary to make a baby.

Of course not to diminish your partner's role in all of this, the second half of that DNA comes from his sperm. And in the process we know as " fertilization", when these two genetic forces combine, the miracle of life is created.

But long before any of this can occur, a series of timely biochemical events must also take place. Orchestrated by a series of hormones designed to help eggs develop, grow, and achieve ovulation , they are the catalyst that ultimately allows your egg to meet with your partner's sperm so that fertilization *can* take place.

While some of these hormones are manufactured inside your ovaries, and others are released by your brain, or stimulated by the release of brain chemical signals, together they work to make pregnancy possible.

The hormones that jump-start the conception process are:

> **FSH - Follicle Stimulating Hormone** : Secreted by the pituitary, a tiny gland located inside your brain, the job of FSH is to send a signal to your ovaries to produce an egg. Indeed, while every woman is born with a lifetime supply of egg follicles (estimates are there are about 400,000 follicles inside your ovaries from the time you are born) without stimulation from FSH, they would never mature into an egg.

> **LH - Luteinizing Hormone** : Also secreted by your pituitary gland, this hormone instructs your matured egg to leave the ovary in the process known as ovulation, and directs it to travel down your fallopian tube where it can meet with your partner's sperm so that fertilization can occur.

Collectively these two hormones are known as "gonadotropins".

While there is some FSH and LH in your body at all times, a significant amount is released during the first half of your menstrual cycle – when your egg is maturing and developing – followed by a dropping off of both hormones after ovulation. To help orchestrate the timing of this rise and fall is a third hormone:

> **GRH or Gonadotropin Releasing Hormone:** Secreted by the hypothalamus (a tiny gland located just above your pituitary) the job of GRH is to direct the release of the proper amounts of FSH and LH into your bloodstream at *the proper time.*

There are also two additional hormones that complete the female reproductive process - and are also intrinsic to getting pregnant.

The first is **estrogen.** Manufactured primarily inside your ovaries, estrogen rises and falls in coordination with brain hormones to help orchestrate egg production and release, and begin to prepare your uterus to receive your fertilized egg. A surge in estrogen around the time of ovulation or egg release also provides more vaginal lubrication. This can increase your desire for sex, and help your partner's sperm travel more easily through your vagina and cervix.

The second is **progesterone.** It's manufactured by the corpus luteum - the shell that an ovulated egg leaves behind. Working in consort with estrogen, progesterone is what helps to prepare your uterus to receive a fertilized egg, and it helps that egg to be nourished and to grow.

How Pregnancy Occurs

At the start of each monthly menstrual cycle, your GRH messengers sense that your estrogen levels are low – a sign that says you are not pregnant. This, in turn, sends a message to step up the production of FSH , which is necessary to stimulate the growth of a new egg.

As FSH surges through your bloodstream, many follicles inside your ovary begin to develop. As days pass, however, only one follicle pulls ahead of the rest in growth and development. Eventually it becomes your "egg of the month" – the one that will be released and available for fertilization. At the same time, however, your egg's rapid growth spurt causes your ovaries to produce more estrogen, and the level rises quite quickly and dramatically. This rise serves two purposes. First, it helps stimulate the lining of your uterus to thicken, in anticipation of receiving a fertilized egg. But more importantly, when estrogen levels reach a specific, predetermined level this signals your brain that your egg has matured and is ready to be released.

To make that happen, your brain releases LH – which as you remember is the hormone which prompts your newly developed egg to pop from your ovary in a process known as "ovulation".

As soon as this happens, the shell which housed your egg turns into a tiny gland known as the corpus luteum, and begins producing progesterone.

Together with estrogen – which is still surging – these two hormones begin creating a spongy nest of blood vessels inside your uterus. Once your egg is fertilized - and becomes an embryo - it travels down your fallopian tube and lands in your uterus, where, if the lining is strong enough, it will attach and begin to grow.

That same spongy lining eventually becomes the "womb" that "nurtures " your embryo with nourishment from your body so that it grows into a strong and healthy baby.

To ensure that this nourishment phase continues – not only now, but throughout your pregnancy - both estrogen and progesterone levels remain high. This in turn signals your brain to keep FSH and LH production at a minimum – which also prevents any new egg follicles from being stimulated into growth and development. This is also why your menstrual cycle stops during pregnancy, and why you *can't* get pregnant again *while* you are pregnant !

If, however, no fertilization takes place, still one more chemical message is sent to your brain - this one designed to signal a rapid drop in both estrogen and progesterone. It is , in fact, this rapid drop that causes the spongy lining inside your uterus to immediately break down and be shed. This shedding process becomes the basis of your menstrual bleed.

Once that bleeding stops – within about 7 days – your body is once again ready to start a new cycle : You prepare, grow and release a new egg and another chance for conception occurs.

Introducing Sperm & Egg

Although this finely tuned biochemical and hormonal network is intrinsic to getting pregnant, none of this would matter if your egg could not hook up with your partner's sperm. And the fact that it does has a lot more to do with science than "chance".

Indeed, the preparation for this momentous event begins the moment your egg matures. When it does, petal-like fingers that sit at the far end of your fallopian tube reach up and begin massaging your ovary, creating a kind of suction that gently coaxes your egg to pop from its shell and slide into the portion of your fallopian tube connected to your ovary. This long, narrow corridor which leads directly to your uterus is actually the place where sperm and egg meet and conception occurs.

And, if the timing is right, while your egg is getting ready to be released, your partner's sperm is swimming within your cervical mucus, through your vaginal canal, into your cervix and up into your fallopian tube from the opposite direction. How exactly does the sperm know where to go? First, your cervical mucus offers some direction, helping to guide sperm in the right direction.

But one of the newest discoveries made about the reproductive process is that the head of each sperm contains a kind of biochemical "radar" designed to pick up hormonal signals from a developing egg. In a kind of biochemical "come hither" flirt, your egg silently calls out to your partner's sperm - and his sperm responds by rapidly swimming forward through your reproductive system.

By the time your egg pops from it's shell and is ovulated, that silent calling is so strong, it acts almost like a magnet, pulling as many sperm as possible to it's side.

But before pregnancy can occur, one of your partner's sperm must penetrate and enter that egg – the step that allows your DNA to combine with his and begin to form your baby.

To help make this happen, the head of each sperm - called the "acrosome" - releases a substance designed to break down the outside shell of your egg . And while all the sperm are competing for the same chance to be "the one" that gets inside, much like your mate who worked the hardest to win your heart, generally one sperm works a little harder and a little faster than all the rest, enabling the entry process to begin.

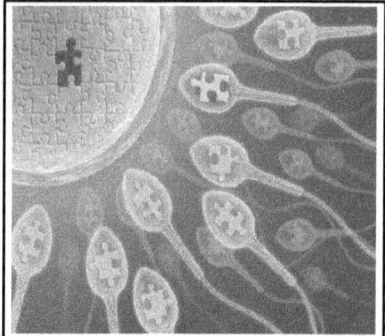

As your egg matures and grows it sends out a silent signal to sperm that fertilization time is nearing. Your partner's sperm picks up that silent signal and responds by swimming quickly through your reproductive system in an effort to reach your egg in time !

Then, much like supportive teammates on the baseball field, as soon as that sperm begins the penetration process, the others step back and begin rooting for the "home run".

To facilitate this, each of the other sperm stops their "drilling" process and pulls away from the egg – thus giving the "lead sperm" a chance to gain entry. Once it does, the others swim away and within a few days, die off and are bio-chemically dissolved by the body.

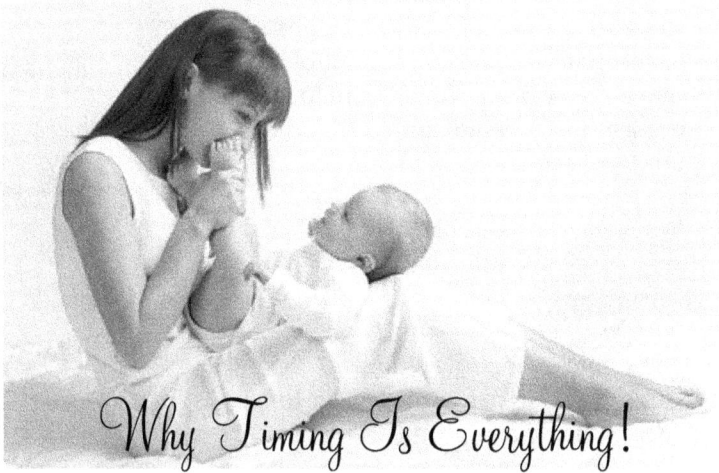

Why Timing Is Everything!

While it may seem that all this activity can pretty much happen any time sperm and egg are in the same place at the same time, the truth is, when it comes to getting pregnant, *timing is everything.*

And by this I mean that in order for conception to occur, your partner's sperm must meet up with your egg no later than 24 hours after it leaves your ovary. This is because the opportunity for fertilization is good for a "limited time only"!

Indeed, while your egg may not carry an obvious expiration date, the truth is, it is only viable – or able to be fertilized – for approximately 12 to 24 hours after ovulation. After that time it begins to break down and disintegrate, so that fertilization cannot occur, or if it does, that "union" usually isn't healthy, and can often result in a miscarriage.

Sperm, on the other hand, have a much longer "shelf life". They can remain alive and ready to fertilize an egg for up to 5 days after they leave a man's body. While this may seem a little unfair, it actually gives you the "home court" advantage! How? Because sperm *can* live longer, that means they can be in your body, ready and waiting for your egg to be ovulated and arrive!

In fact, one of the biggest "conception" mistakes couples make is waiting until ovulation occurs to become intimate and attempt pregnancy.

While it's still possible, if his sperm are just a little bit slow in "swimming" towards your fallopian tube, or if minor biochemical snafus diminish the "guiding" signal from egg-to-sperm, then waiting until ovulation day to have sex will likely mean the egg-sperm "hook up" simply occurs too late in the game for a viable conception to occur.

Fertility Tip: To get pregnant fast be sure to make love beginning 3 days before you expect to ovulate and continue daily until one day past ovulation.

So, in this respect, the number one easiest way to insure conception is to begin making love once daily, up to 5 days before ovulation is expected to occur. (If you're not sure how to tell when ovulation is approaching you can download our FREE E-book on 6 ways to predict ovulation. You will find the link at : www.GettingPregnantNow.org

Once you know when you are ovulating, having sex during this time frame gives your partner's sperm plenty of opportunity to make their way to your fallopian tube and be there, ready and waiting, for your egg to make it's "entrance".

This, in turn, allows the fertilization process to begin as quickly as possible, with an egg that is at the "peak" of perfection.

Ultimately this creates the "optimum" circumstance for a quick, easy and healthy pregnancy to occur!

When Pregnancy Doesn't Happen...

If you're like many of my patients, right about now you may be wondering why making love at the 'right time" doesn't automatically lead to pregnancy *every time* – and why it can take so long to get pregnant.

First, it's important to remember that no matter how much we have learned about the "science" of conception there is still some indefinable "magic" involved. Indeed, even when all conditions are right for pregnancy – a healthy egg is made and ovulated at the right time, and a hearty group of healthy sperm is ready and waiting to pounce – it's still Mother Nature who has the last word! This is why it can some couples take up to 12 months to get pregnant naturally - even when no problem exists.

But that said, there are also a number of biological, even medical reasons why conception does not occur each and every time you have intercourse – *even at the right time of the month.*

Among the most common is that you won't necessarily ovulate an egg every single month. While this is less likely to happen when you are in your teens and early 20's (one reason that young women seem to get pregnant so easily) a slight slow down in ovulation can begin as early as your mid-twenties. This is particularly true if you have a full, multi-tasking life, a less than optimal diet, and your days are filled with stress - all factors that can greatly influence egg production and release.

Moreover, these same factors can also impact sperm production as well - and certainly ,at least 50% of the time conception problems are related to male factors. This includes a reduction in the amount of sperm being produced and released, as well as a reduction in the quality of that sperm - each of which can make getting pregnant more difficult. Because these problems are so often the result of lifestyle factors, particularly diet, I hope you will

share some of the fertility food secrets you learn in this book with
your partner! That said, there are also a number of more specific
reproductive issues that can interfere with conception and make
getting pregnant harder than it has to be. Taking a few more
moments to learn a bit about these problems - and the way in which
diet can help - will ultimately allow you to make better use of
everything included in this book.

Women, Hormones & Getting Pregnant

Among the most common conception-related problems in women
is a hormone imbalance, usually between estrogen and
progesterone. Depending on the severity of the imbalance it can
cause anything from a temporary disruption in ovulation, to
completely throwing your menstrual cycle - and your ability to get
pregnant - completely off track.

 While any number of factors can cause a hormone imbalance to
occur - including medical conditions such as thyroid disorder - for
the vast majority of women problems are a result of common, every
day influences. These include stress, fatigue, too much or too little
exercise, or most especially, poor diet and nutrition.

For some of you, certainly a tell-tale sign of a hormone imbalance is
raging bouts of PMS   (pre menstrual syndrome),   that can
sometimes occur for up to 10 days during every cycle.

Another symptom can be irregular periods - you consistently miss
cycles completely, or your cycles are erratic , both in length and in
terms of the time between each period.

That said, just as often small, sub-clinical hormone imbalances,
some too slight to even be measured - can also exist, making it
difficult to conceive. And when any of these conditions exist, most
assuredly a change in diet can make a huge difference in getting
your cycle back on track.

Infertility In Younger Women

While many women associate infertility with "older" women, the truth is that today, more and more "younger" women are having problems getting pregnant. While for some it's clearly hormonal disorders at work, for many others, problems are a bit more serious.

Indeed, among the most common medical problem causing infertility in younger women is the menstrual-related disorder known as "endometriosis" .

Here, tiny bits of uterine tissue meant to leave the body as menstrual blood instead travel from the uterus and land on other organs in the pelvic region. Once there they take hold and begin to form lesions. As these lesions grown, they can form blockages within the reproductive system that, without treatment, can block conception.

Another problem that is also impacting more and more younger women is PCOS - short for poly cystic ovarian syndrome. In this disorder the ovaries manufacture eggs but most times cannot release them, so ovulation rarely occurs.

While it might seems as if this is a problem within the ovaries, more recently doctors have discovered it's actually a condition that is related to blood sugar . Indeed, hormones involved in clearing sugar from the blood, including insulin, are part of a finely tuned network that also plays a role in reproduction. So when this system goes awry it can also impact the ovaries - and again, without treatment pregnancy becomes difficult, or even impossible.

In both conditions, medications can be extremely effective. But studies show that diet can also play a key role in not only controlling symptoms, but also in helping to encourage pregnancy in those who try. And to this end throughout this book you will find some special advice and suggestions for foods that can have an especially important influence on both these disorders.

Getting Pregnant After 35

Still one more condition than can interfere with conception is, quite simply, your age! Indeed, while your face and your body may look 25, it's your ovaries that "give away" how many candles are really on your birthday cake! That's because as a woman ages, so do the follicles inside her ovary. And as they do, fewer and fewer of them have the ability to "ripen" into an egg that is healthy enough for fertilization.

Now if you're thinking this is something that only happens to women approaching menopause, guess again. Indeed in many women eggs begin to show signs of age as early as their early thirties. More importantly, a number of lifestyle factors - including smoking, drinking alcohol and especially a poor diet - can contribute to the "aging " process, reducing chances for conception much earlier than you might think.

The good news here: Studies show that small but simple changes in diet and lifestyle can have, perhaps the most impact of all in this group. Indeed, not only can the nutrients found in certain foods help slow down the aging process of your ovaries, in some instances they have the power to protect and even rejuvenate the entire reproductive process, so that you can get pregnant naturally, even after age 40.

Of course no diet is going to reverse menopause - or kick start ovulation in women that are long past their reproductive prime.

Still, for those of you in the middle years - between 40 and 50 - with or without medical treatments, I have seen diet have some pretty miraculous results in terms of encouraging conception - even in women who were told by other doctors that donor eggs were their only chance! Indeed, if you are over 35 and trying to conceive, be sure to follow the food plan in this book as closely as you can - I promise you that doing so will really pay off!

Explaining "Unexplained Infertility"

While the problems we just discussed are among the most common reason why pregnancy is delayed, they are not the only ones. Indeed, for a growing number of couples - even those who visit fertility clinics - the single most common problem being diagnosed today is a condition known as "unexplained infertility".

In fact, it may surprise you to know that this is actually the most common diagnosis made in fertility clinics worldwide.

But what, exactly, does it mean? Essentially 'unexplained infertility" is an indication that while both partner's reproductive systems appear to be working "right", there is a constellation of small, sometimes "sub-clinical" glitches in the baby-making system that come together to prevent pregnancy from occurring. This can be a slight hormonal imbalance in one or both partners, or as is often the case, the result of one or more environmental and lifestyle factors that are preventing the reproductive system from functioning optimally. Indeed, during my 30 plus years of experience treating infertile couples in American and in Europe, the single most important factor I have seen make a difference *is diet*. In fact, I have personally treated a great number of couples who went from "unexplained infertility" to parenthood in less than a year by doing nothing more than changing what they eat and living a bit more of a healthy lifestyle.

In fact, if you fall into any of the categories we just discussed - from irregular ovulation to hormonal imbalances, from endometriosis to PCOS, or if your partner is affected by less than optimal sperm, then I am quite certain that a change in diet will be your answer as well. In addition to my own personal studies and observations gathered from treating thousands of patients throughout the years, there are also excellent studies to show that by adding certain foods into your diet - and eliminating others - you can not only help optimize hormone production and ovulation (regardless of your age), but also create healthier eggs, and ultimately, a healthier baby. The same is true for many sperm related problems which, in some cases, respond even more quickly to simple diet and lifestyle changes.

Getting Pregnant Fast: Now You Can!

Of course it would be wrong to suggest that a diet alone can solve all fertility problems - because it just isn't true. While I do believe it can make a huge difference in every couple trying to conceive, for some, it may work best in conjunction with medical treatments - particularly when a physiological problem -such as blocked fallopian tubes or an inability to make eggs- is preventing you from getting pregnant.

For this reason, my personal advice is that if you are under age 35 and trying for more than a year to get pregnant, or over age 35 and trying for six months or longer to conceive, then certainly follow this diet - but also talk to your doctor about some baseline fertility tests, for you and your partner. Odds are that for most of you, no serious problems will be found. But knowing that for sure will help free you from worry that there "might" be something wrong - and reducing this stress may help encourage your fertility as well.

And in the event that a problem *is* discovered, fear not! Today there are a multitude of new and easy options able to help you! For those of you who want to learn more about these options we have detailed all the most pertinent findings in our best selling book "Getting Pregnant:What You Need to Know Now" and on our website, www.GettingPregnantNow.org.

For right now, however, I invite you to sit back, relax, put your feet up and read on to discover how to eat the most delicious foods ever – and get pregnant fast! Whether you are in your 20's and simply looking to increase your odds of a natural conception, or you've been trying for a while to conceive, I can promise you that the secrets in this book can and will make a difference in your life!

CHAPTER TWO:

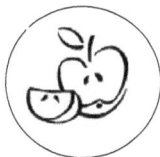

Super Protein Fertility Power!

Choose the right type of protein & watch your fertility soar!

For many years. I , and many fertility experts, have been telling patients about a powerful fertility secret - a food group that can have an enormous power to encourage and enhance fertility in all women.

That food group is protein. Found in abundance in foods such as fish, poultry and lean red meat as well as in beans, soy and many varieties of nuts, studies have shown, and I have seen within my own patient population, the power of protein to enhance fertility.

Indeed, in my previous books, and throughout years of counseling fertility patients, I have always recommended increasing protein intake as a way of enhancing fertility.

How, exactly, does protein accomplish this? The impact of these foods is primarily on ovulation.

In fact, studies show that when protein intake is high, ovulation occurs more regularly. Conversely, drop your protein intake too low and you will likely see a disruption in your menstrual cycle, sometimes to the point where ovulation stops completely, so there is no chance of getting pregnant - at least not until ovarian function is restored.

Also important: There are isolated studies suggesting that dietary protein can impact blood sugar and increase sensitivity to insulin, which, as you will discover a little later in this book, has a direct link to ovulation.

Moreover when you do get pregnant, increasing your protein intake is even more important, for you and your baby. According to the American College of Obstetricians and Gynecologists, consuming an adequate amount of protein during pregnancy can increase your developing baby's birth weight - and that can lead to a healthier baby overall.

Not All Fertility Proteins Are Alike!

When it comes to choosing what type of protein to eat, you have several options to consider. I have always personally believed that lean red meat, followed by white meat poultry and fish are among the best sources of protein if you are trying to get pregnant.

That said, some of the newer research shows that while the protein content of these foods is still important for fertility, a few other factors, including certain inflammatory compounds and fat content found in red meat and mercury levels in fish, can counter some of the good effects these foods provide.

For this reason I now recommend that you still eat these foods, but to do so in moderation, and to eat smaller portions.

So, for example, you eat up to 12 ounces of fish a week and gain all the benefits, without worrying about the risks. Similarly, you can feel good about eating 3 to 3.5 ounces of red meat 3 to 4 times a week without fear. As long as you remove the skin from your poultry, you can safely gain the fertility-boosting effects of it's protein content, and you can eat it in any amount.

How To Give Your Fertility An Extra Protein Boost!

While for some women these high protein foods may provide enough of a boost to keep fertility on track, if you want to increase your chances for getting pregnant even further, you should consider adding some additional protein sources to your diet - particularly in the form of vegetable proteins found in foods like beans and nuts.

In fact, these are some of the foods that were recently targeted as very helpful in a major study on ovulation conducted by researchers at Harvard University. According to their findings, women with the highest intake of plant proteins had fewer ovulatory problems overall, compared to women who ate mostly animal based proteins.

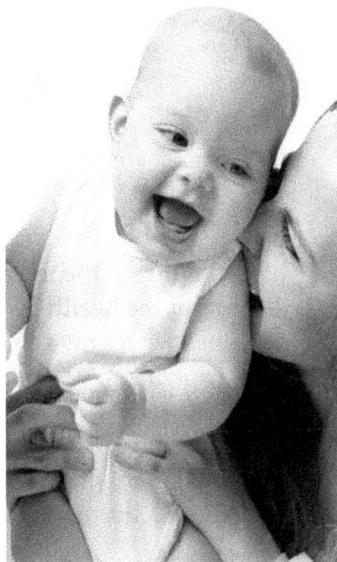

More specifically, the Harvard study found that when total calories were the same, women who added just one serving per week of plant based protein to their diet - including beans, tofu, soybeans, peanuts or other nuts - appeared to garner protection against many types of ovulatory related fertility problems.

Treats you might never think of as a "fertility food" such as a grilled steak or a cheeseburger can actually help you pregnant. That's because they are high in protein - which is good for ovulation! The key is to eat them in moderation.

Choose Your Plant Proteins Wisely

While I agree in theory with the Harvard findings, particularly in terms of the health benefits of increasing your intake of plant proteins, where my recommendations differ is in the source of those proteins.

More specifically, I believe that consuming a large amount of soy-based plant proteins is not a good good idea, particularly if you have a a hormone imbalance that is affecting your fertility.

Now certainly, if you spend even a little time on the Internet researching the impact of soy on fertility, you are likely to find a number of sites filled with anecdotal stories of women who have regulated their menstrual cycles and improved their fertility profile by consuming large amounts of soy. Some, in fact, have claimed that soy encourages egg production and release as effectively fertility drugs such as Clomid, with the effects credited to the plant estrogens found in soy.

But as encouraging and well meaning as these anecdotal reports are, I feel I must caution you about what a number of medical studies, other than the new Harvard study, have to say on this subject.

Indeed, a good deal of the research has found that soy either has no impact on ovulation, or it has a slightly detrimental effect. When this occurs, it may actually reduce fertility and make it harder for some women to get pregnant.

- In one meta-analysis published in the Journal of Nutrition in 2002, researchers pointed to a number of a studies which found that increased soy intake frequently resulted in a longer menstrual cycle and a decrease in estrogen, progesterone and other biochemicals necessary for conception.

- In a study published a few years earlier in the American Journal of Clinical Nutrition, researchers found that a diet high in soy actually suppressed both FSH and LH, two key hormones necessary for egg production and ovulation.

- More recently a study published in the European Journal of Nutrition found that soy foods had no impact on fertility and offered no increase in pregnancy odds.

Of course all these studies conflict somewhat with the new Harvard findings which reported women who ate a diet high in soy were protected against some forms of infertility.

So, where does the truth about soy lie? At the moment I don't think anyone knows for certain. And ultimately it is my guess that it may turn out that soy foods are helpful for some women and not for others. For right now, however, I would say that if you already know you have an ovulation problem and that your ovaries are not making enough estrogen, then it would be wise to increase your intake of soy protein.

To get pregnant faster, try making love on your birthday!
A study published in the Japanese medical journal Gynaekologe reports that in some women fertility is season-sensitive increasing around the time of their birthday !

Conversely, if you are ovulating on time, and you're pretty sure that your ovaries are functioning normally, then my recommendation is to go light and easy on the soy rich foods, simply because you don't need that extra estrogen stimulation.

If you're not sure whether or not you have ovulation issues or even a hormonal problem, then certainly it's okay to add some soy foods to your diet because they are a good source of plant protein, but do so in moderation.

In fact, my overall philosophy is that, when in doubt, follow the principals upon which all sound nutritional programs are based and vary your diet so that it includes a wide variety of nutritional foods - including protein from a variety of sources. This includes both plant and animal based proteins.

In this way you and your fertility will reap the benefits of everything these foods have to offer!

The New Fertility Protein

If you're like to add more plant-based proteins to your diet but want to limit your soy intake, you might want to consider another high-protein legume known as "lupin".

Grown in Australia but now being milled worldwide into flours for bread, rolls, and other baked goods, lupin is not only high in plant proteins (much higher than soy!) but it also contains significant fiber, which as you will discover later in this book can have a positive and important impact on your fertility.

In fact, with just a little creativity on your part, I can promise you will discover that the foods which can boost your fertility can also satisfy your taste buds and your appetite.

And don't forget that in many instances your partner's health and his fertility can benefit from these same foods. So, be sure to share your "healthy baby" meals together as often as possible!

Also remember to use the Fertility Food Guide featured later in this book to expand your menu options by combining protein with lots of fertility-boosting fruits, vegetables and whole grains, which you will learn more about in the chapters to come!

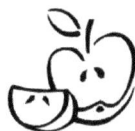

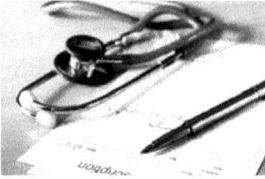

YOUR FERTILITY FOOD PRESCRIPTION:

Protein:

- *3 servings of fresh fish per week.*
- *2 servings of either red meat or poultry per week.*
- *3 servings of nuts per week.*
- *3 to 5 servings of any plant based protein per week including nuts.*

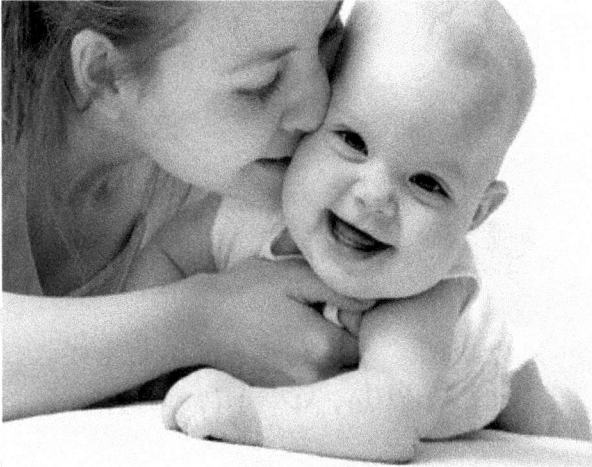

Want To Get Pregnant Fast?
Try A Vacation In The Sun!

Studies show that women who live in warmer climates with more sun exposure have fewer fertility problems! The key appears to be Vitamin D which your body makes from the sun. When D levels are high, fertility can thrive!

Want to get pregnant in winter & can't get away? Try Vitamin D supplements.

You'll need about 1,000 units daily .

CHAPTER THREE:

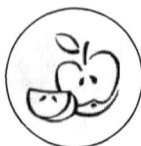

Breads, Muffins, Pasta & Pregnancy: What You Need To Know!

If you're like many of my patients, in the days just prior to your menstrual cycle food takes on a much bigger and more important meaning! I'm talking about food cravings and for many of you I know that this includes an almost insatiable urge for one group of foods above all others. If you haven't already guessed, this group is known as carbohydrates.

And while most of you probably know this is a broad category that includes foods such as fruits, vegetables and grains, I'm guessing that for most you, spinach and cauliflower is not high on your pre-menstrual "must eat" list.

Indeed, for most women, the very term "carbohydrates" is focused on the other foods in this category: Bread, pasta, cake, cookies, puddings and pies!

Call them comfort foods, happiness foods, even *fun foods*, but if you're like most of my patients, these are the items you can't seem to get enough of, beginning around the middle of your menstrual cycle.

Well the fact that you do crave them during the time when you are most likely to get pregnant is one of the first clues that carbohydrates might have a link to getting pregnant.

And in fact, they do. But if you're thinking that all you need do is load up on jelly sandwiches and chocolate-chip cookies to get pregnant, it's time to step away from the fridge and listen up!

Indeed, while some carbohydrates can definitely encourage your chances of getting pregnant, others can hamper or even completely block all chances of conception.

Discovering which carbohydrates fall on which side of the fertility fence is actually the first secret to understanding how these foods can help you get pregnant faster!

Carbohydrates & Conception: Don't Make This Mistake!

As many of you already know, most of the so-called "comfort carbohydrates" - foods like cake, pie, cookies, muffins and macaroni - fall under a category known as "simple carbs".

And the fact that they earned this name is no accident. Indeed they are called "simple" because once eaten, they don't require any complicated biochemistry in order to be digested.

In fact, almost immediately after eating a simple carb - like a cookie or a piece of white bread - your body quickly begins to break it down into "simple sugars". These are molecules which are rapidly absorbed into your bloodstream.

The type of carbohydrate you choose can make a huge difference in how well your reproductive hormones function.
If you choose wisely - you can satisfy your carb cravings and boost your fertility !

For this reason "simple carbs" are known to have a "high glycemic load". What's this? In simple terms it means they have the capacity to release lots of sugar into the bloodstream quickly.

But while these "simple carbs" may be the foods you are most familiar with, they only make up one-half of the carbohydrate story. Because falling under the heading of "carbohydrates", are a whole other category of foods. These include fruits, vegetables, and whole grains, such as whole wheat, oats and rye. Together they make up the sub-group known as "complex carbohydrates".

They are called "complex" because it not only requires more effort to break them down and digest them, but also because they require more steps before they can release sugar into your bloodstream. Indeed, because these foods release sugar so slowly, they are know to have a "Low Glycemic Load.

So, what does all this have to do with getting pregnant? Well the answer to that question can be found in understanding a little bit more about insulin - the key hormone involved in metabolizing these foods.

Insulin And Your Fertility: What You Must Know

Manufactured by your pancreas, (an organ located smack in the middle of your upper tummy region), the job of insulin is to clear sugar from your blood and carry it to your cells. Here the sugars are stored, and later used for energy by every organ and muscle in your body.

As such, soon after blood sugar levels start to rise, your pancreas begins pouring out insulin. Turning into a sort of biochemical "door knocker" it is this rise in insulin that signals cells to "open up" and let the sugar in.

Now when you eat small amounts of "simple" carbohydrates, or when you eat them only occasionally, your body does a pretty good job of producing enough insulin to get the sugar-clearing job done. Moreover, when insulin levels aren't maxed out your cells remain very responsive to that "knock on the door."

As such there is no problem getting sugar out of your bloodstream and into your cells. This means you have lots of energy for all the muscles and organs in your body to function at full capacity, including your brain and all the reproductive biochemistry that begins in the brain.

But what happens when you begin to crave, and load-up too many "simple carbs" - particularly over a longer period of time?

First, the more of these foods you eat, the harder your pancreas has to work to pour out enough insulin to remove the sugars from your bloodstream. But even more importantly, the more often that your cells are forced to "answer" insulin's "knock on the door," the less responsive they get. And that means even more insulin is needed to get those cells to "open up" and let the sugar in.

When this occurs a condition known as "insulin resistance" develops. This is not only the precursor to the much more serious type 2 diabetes, for many women it is also the first step on the road to infertility.

For many women, insulin resistance is not just the precursor to type 2 diabetes, it's also the first warning sign of infertility.

The Good News: You can reverse the effects, improve your general health and recharge your fertility, simply by eating the right foods!

Why does this occur? Because insulin is a hormone, it's production and release is part of a finely tuned network of balanced hormonal activity, some of which is involved in egg production and release.

And so, when your body is being continually forced to produce large amounts of insulin for a long period of time as is the case when you eat a diet high in "simple" carbohydrates - the hormonal network necessary for conception is disrupted in a number of key ways.

Among the first things that happens is an increase in the production of androgens. These are male hormones including testosterone. Under normal conditions testosterone is produced by your ovaries, but only in very tiny amounts. However, when insulin levels are consistently high, it sends a message to your ovaries to step up testosterone production, while slowing down or even stopping estrogen production.

Once this happens it dramatically affects both your ability to make a healthy egg or to release it from your ovary. As such a temporary form of infertility occurs.

Moreover, if left to continue on long enough some women stop ovulation completely and a longer, more difficult form of infertility takes hold. This can often be the case for women with an insulin-related fertility disorder known as PCOS - poly cystic ovarian syndrome. In this condition eggs are trapped inside the ovary and cannot be ovulated at all.

But even if you don't have this problem, eating a diet high in simple carbohydrates can still cause enough of an impact on your body so that a form of insulin resistance occurs. When it does, not only is it harder to get pregnant, but without treatment it can be almost impossible for some women.

And in fact that is exactly what a group of Harvard researchers found when they analyzed data from a massive nationwide Nurses Health Project.

The study, which involved over 18,000 women found that those who consumed a diet high in quick burning "simple" carbohydrates were 92% more likely to experience ovulatory-related infertility than women who ate less of these foods.

Indeed, in some women, continually snacking on foods like white bread, pasta, cookies, potatoes and white rice didn't just hamper their ability to get pregnant quickly, it actually blocked them from getting pregnant at all!

Perhaps more importantly, this finding appeared to hold true even after the researchers took into consideration factors that impact the result - such as age, smoking, and the consumption of animal fat, which is another food related to fertility that you'll learn more about a little later.

> *In one study women who continually snacked on cakes & cookies didn't just have a harder time getting pregnant - they could not conceive at all! Likewise, women who consumed a diet high in simple carbohydrates were 92% more likely to be infertile.*

The Carbohydrates That Can Help You Get Pregnant Fast!

If you're like many of my patients you might be thinking that the best way to get pregnant fast is to simply stop eating all carbohydrates no matter your food cravings! But that would be a big mistake. Why?

Because what researchers also discovered is that some carbohydrates are definitely necessary to promote fertility and some can even help you get pregnant faster!

Remember you read earlier that not all carbohydrates are alike? Indeed, the Nurses Health Study also found that women who ate diets high in "complex carbohydrates" - those slow burning carbs we talked about earlier - decreased their risk of ovulatory problems and got pregnant faster!

This finding dovetails perfectly with previous research showing that most slow burning carbohydrates are also high in fiber, a type non-nutritive compound that also helps to keep blood sugar balanced while it also works to pull heart-harming cholesterol from your blood.

Indeed, the American Dietetic Association has confirmed that fiber is an essential element for controlling blood sugar as well as helping to control weight - two factors that play an important role in fertility.

So, while it's clear that your body and your fertility need carbohydrates in order to function properly, not all carbohydrates have the same effect.

But, by reducing your intake of "simple" carbohydrates (like white rice, potatoes and anything made of white flour) and increasing your intake of complex carbohydrates (like whole grain cereals and plenty of fruits and vegetables) you will increase your chance of getting pregnant quicker and easier.

Not coincidentally the same foods that are good for fertility are also good for your heart - and may help you live a longer and a healthier life - which will definitely benefit your baby as well!

Later in this book you'll find my Fertility Food Guide - which includes not only a list of the foods most likely to encourage fertility, but also the "glycemic load index" of each of those foods. Using those numbers as a guide it will be easy to choose the carbohydrates that can benefit your fertility most.

So, does this mean you have to cut out all the "simple" carbs you love and crave? Definitely not! The key, however is to eat them in smaller portions and to balance their effects by combining them with foods high in protein, some "healthy" fats (which you'll read more about a little later in the book) and fiber - all of which can slow down sugar release. So, for example, by making a pan of brownies using whole wheat flour and adding high protein nuts, you will neutralize some of the impact of the sugars and feed your cravings and your fertility in one delicious dessert!

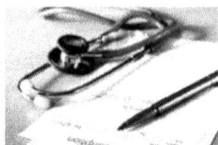

YOUR FERTILITY FOOD PRESCRIPTION:

Carbohydrates

- Eat at least 20 or more grams of fiber daily.

- Make certain a whole grain is the first ingredient in all breads and muffins.

- Choose whole fruits in place of fruit juices.

- Include at last one fruit with your breakfast.

- Add more beans to your diet (they're loaded with complex carbs and vegetable proteins).

- Switch to whole wheat pasta.

- Choose a high fiber breakfast cereal such as bran flakes or oatmeal.

- Reduce your intake of "simple" carbohydrates such as cakes, cookies, breads and pies made with white flour. Whenever possible, substitute carbs made with whole grains.

CHAPTER FOUR:

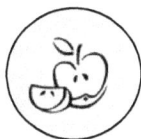

The Fruits Vegetables, Nuts & Seeds with Amazing Fertility Powers!

There is perhaps no greater culinary sensation then biting into a juicy ripe peach on a hot summer's day – or a crisp red apple when there's a nip of fall in the air!

The same can be said for a handful of nuts – or basket of whole grain croissants. Indeed, dipping into Mother Nature's bounty can offer taste sensations that can be hard to beat.

But eating these – and other fruits , vegetables, nuts and seeds, offers more than just a taste treat.

In fact, an abundance of medical studies now show that when it comes to getting pregnant, frequent dips into Mother Nature's bounty can be a wonderful and tasty way to boost fertility and get pregnant faster!

How and why can these foods help you?

As you just read in the previous chapter on fertility foods, fruits and vegetables fall into a nutritional category known as "carbohydrates".

Since most are "slow burning" *complex* carbohydrates, they can easily offer you all the blood sugar and hormone balancing benefits of other foods in this same group, including whole grains.

But from both a general health - and a pregnancy - standpoint, the benefits of adding fruits, vegetables, nuts and seeds into your daily diet goes far beyond simply protecting you from insulin resistance and related fertility problems. How?

Certain fruits & vegetables have a specific effect on fertility, influencing the hormone activity necessary for getting pregnant fast!

First, these foods are a powerful source of both healthy fiber and many of the key vitamins that impact fertility - including Vitamins C, B complex, E and folate.

But there are also additional, equally important ways in which natural compounds found in these foods can have some direct effects on your fertility, influencing not only hormone activity but also the growth, development and ovulation of healthy eggs.

For all these reasons I'm devoting an entire chapter to filling you in on the most important ways that these natural fertility boosters can help you get pregnant faster and easier!

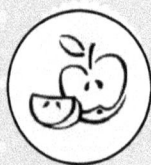

The Awesome Power of Fruits & Veggies

While almost every fruit and vegetable on the planet offers at least one or more specific health benefit, when it comes to getting pregnant perhaps the greatest advantage involves protecting you from " free radicals ".

This is a type of molecule that forms via exposure to certain lifestyle factors. These can include a diet high in saturated fat, exposure to tobacco smoke - including second hand smoke, chemical toxins from pesticides, household cleaners or even some cosmetics and skin care items, or even overexposure to the sun.

But what exactly is a "free radical" and how can it harm your fertility? Essentially, a "free radical" is a type of adulterated oxygen molecule. Indeed unlike a "normal" oxygen molecule, which contains a pair of tiny particles called "electrons", a free radical contains only one electron. And because of that they are always on a mission to find the mate. And while this may sound like a bit of "science romance" , in truth, the search for it's missing electron is where all the problems related to fertility usually begin.

Because in order to find their electron mate, free radicals act like tiny molecular assassins, targeting the outer membranes of

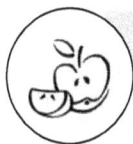

While the vitamins found in fruits & veggies are important, their real fertility power is in their antioxidant potential -the ability to protect your body from factors that harm fertility !

healthy cells in an effort to steal their electrons. In a process known as "lipid oxidation" the free radicals cause a kind of oxidative stress that begins to damage the outer protective membranes of every cell it attacks. Moreover, every time a free radical attacks a cell it causes another free radical to be generated.

Eventually, if not put in check, free radical production can reign out of control, and in the process begin to destroy that outer coating of every cell they come in contact with.

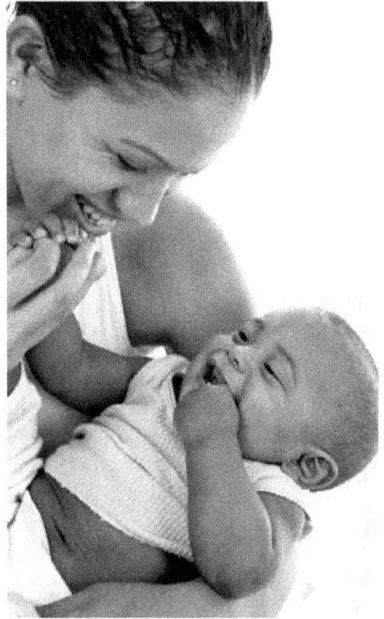

Once this occurs, it literally opens the door allowing the free radical to get inside, where it can immediately begin to attack and alter the factors necessary for healthy cell function. This includes damaging the DNA – the very essence of every cell in your body.

Indeed, when enough DNA damage to enough cells occurs the stage is set for a host of diseases to develop, including cancer, diabetes, Alzheimer's, Parkinson's and yes, some forms of infertility.

Indeed, one study published in the Journal of Human Reproduction in 2007 suggests that oxidative cell damage has such a direct and dramatic impact on a woman's fertility that when large enough numbers of cells are involved, the ensuing damage can make it impossible for pregnancy to occur.

In another study published in the same journal in 2008, doctors found that when the follicular fluid surrounding a woman's eggs was exposed to oxidative stress her eggs became damaged and were less likely to be fertilized.

But that discovery, it seems, was just the beginning.

Indeed, dozens of studies now show that in one form or another, free radicals and their resulting oxidative stress cause cell damage and impair fertility in a number of ways including :

- Impacting the ability of your eggs to mature and develop.
- Interfering with regular ovulation.
- Causing or exacerbating changes in the lining of the uterus, making it difficult for an embryo to attach and grow and increasing the risk of miscarriage.
- Impacting the lining of the fallopian tubes which in turn can keep sperm from reaching your egg or prevent a fertilized egg from reaching your uterus.
- Creating a hormonal imbalance significant enough to interfere with fertility on a number of different levels.

Most recently, damage from free radicals has been proven to be a significant factor in "unexplained infertility"- one of the most common findings among couples who visit a fertility specialist.

And, it's not just women were who are affected. Indeed, research now shows that male fertility and the production of healthy sperm can also be impacted by free radical damage.

Fruits & Veggies To The Rescue!

While both free radicals and the resulting oxidative stress can have an enormous negative impact on your health and your fertility, it doesn't have to be this way! Indeed, you have the power to change your fertility destiny ...and food can be your strongest defense!

In fact, when it comes to protection from free radical damage, there are perhaps no greater warriors willing to come to your defense than fruits and vegetables!

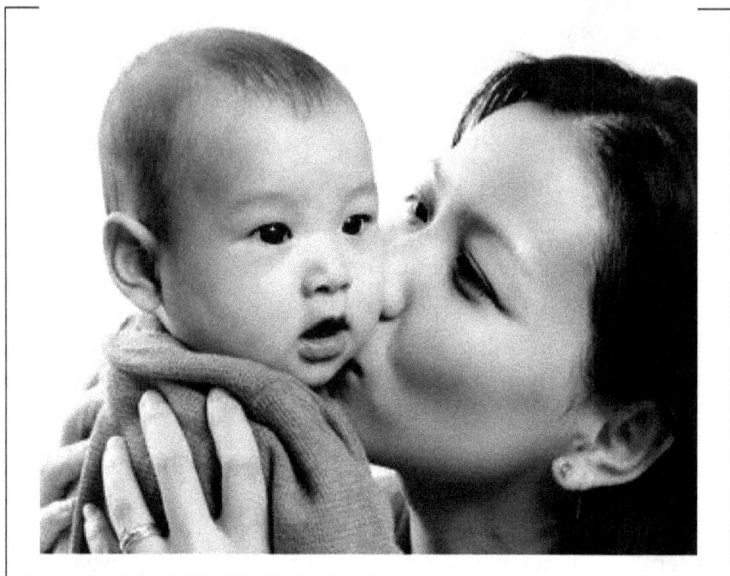

Peaches, plums, apricots, nectarines, broccoli, beans, cabbage and cauliflower are just some of the "fertility soldiers" that go to work every day to help you get pregnant!

How exactly do they do that?

First, they are loaded to the brim with natural compounds known as antioxidants. Much like their name implies an antioxidant is a molecule that protects against " oxidative damage ". How?

Once ingested, antioxidant molecules literally float through your body searching out or "scavenging" free radical molecules. When   they   find them they latch on tight and disarm and disable them, protecting your cells from damage, and preventing new free radicals from forming. With fewer free radicals able to cause damage and fewer free radicals being made, it's easy to see how your health and your fertility can prosper!

In fact, in one study published in the Journal of Human Reproduction in 2008, findings suggested that a diet high in antioxidants can favorably influence not only how quickly and easily an egg can be fertilized, but also whether or not the resulting embryo will survive and thrive or be lost to an early stage miscarriage.

And on this point I can tell you from my own patient population that many women who came to see me believing they could not get pregnant were surprised to discover they had actually been conceiving but losing their conception to early stage miscarriage - so early in fact they did not even know they were pregnant.

So it is indeed comforting to know that a simple change in diet may be all that is necessary to stop the cycle of early miscarriage for many women, and finally allow them to bring a happy, healthy baby into their world!

But it's not just pregnancy loss that's affected by antioxidants. These powerful nutrients also have the ability to neutralize a host of fertility robbing activities and in doing so increase your ability to get pregnant faster as well a help you maintain your good health now and in the future.

But there is still more good news to discover! Indeed, antioxidants are just one component of a complex network of natural compounds known as "phytonutrients". These are natural, health-giving chemicals found in a great abundance in fruits, vegetables, nuts and seeds. And when it comes to boosting fertility, these are among the most powerful natural factors you can find!

So, I invite you to read on and discover how these delicious and nutritious compounds work, and exactly where to find them !

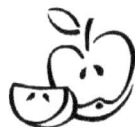

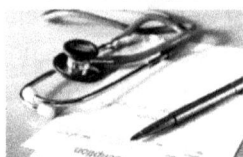

YOUR FERTILITY FOOD PRESCRIPTION

Fruits & Veggies

- Try to eat at least 5 fruits & veggies every day.
- Strive to include both one fruit and one veggie at every meal.
- Remember that the brighter the color of your fruits & veggies the more fertility nutrients you'll be getting.
- Try to eat one red or blue berry daily.
- When you get a craving for a cookie or piece of cake, eat a piece of fruit first; the craving will most likely pass.
- Switch out white potatoes for a high fiber, slower digesting carb such as cauliflower or yams.
- Aim for 3 meals a week that consist solely of fruits, veggies and a high fiber carb .
- When ordering pizza, skip the extra cheese and instead ask for a veggie topping such as broccoli or extra tomatoes.

CHAPTER FIVE

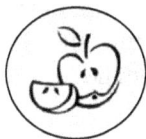

The Secret Nutrients That Help You Get Pregnant Fast!

One of the unique things about plants – of all types – is that they don't possess the same kind of biochemical "warning" system about impending dangers that both humans and animals do.

Indeed, the adrenalin-fueled "fight or flight" response that is genetically programmed into our DNA works to both alert us to danger and help us to escape it. But plants don't have that unique advantage.

Still, Mother Nature didn't leave her beloved plants totally unprotected. They possess a very special kind of natural chemical repair system - a network, in fact, of natural compounds that protects them from harm. At the center of that network are natural chemicals known as "phytonutrients".

Their job is to protect plants from assault by insects, fungus or any environmental threat including the damaging rays of ultra violet light from the sun. And herein lies one clue as to how phytonutrients can help protect you as well.

Because what's really incredible is that from the moment you start eating the fruits and vegetables highest in these protective phytonutrients, you began to garner some of the same protection that Mother Nature bestowed on her beloved plants. Indeed, you not only get the benefit of protection from free radical damage, you also get some of the same cellular repair activity that helps plants to thrive, even under the most adverse of conditions. In fact, all totaled, it's a system that not only stops cellular damage that can harm fertility, but also helps to begin repairing any damage that has already occurred!

In fact, for for many years, researchers believed that the health benefits of eating fruits and vegetables came solely from their vitamin content - specifically the "antioxidant vitamins" such as C, E, and beta carotene. And while they are still considered important for your health and your fertility, in the past decade and particularly in the past five years we have come to recognize that the real protection from fruits and vegetables may actually come not just from vitamins but from their steady supply of phytonutrients.

So how much can these phytonutrients really help you? One recent study shed some new light on just how powerful these compounds are.

In this study researchers intentionally caused severe damage to a strand of DNA - not unlike what might happen to your cells DNA if you were exposed to massive amounts of pollutants.

After the damage had occurred, they treated the broken strand with several different types of phytonutrients, as well as with Vitamin C. The next step involved using a computer to analyze the results and see which factors - the nutrients or the vitamins did best.

The result: The researchers discovered that the combination of phytonutrients used to repair the DNA did a much better, more thorough job than the the Vitamin C alone.

The best news of all: Research now shows these same powerful phytonutrients also have the ability to impact egg development and encourage fertilization. Moreover, it's not just female fertility that can reap the benefits. In research published in the journal Teratogenisis, Carcinogenisis and Mutagenisis researchers found certain phytonutrient compounds were also able to repair damaged sperm, making them better able to fertilize an egg! Since many lifestyle factors can cause a man to manufacture damaged sperm - including smoking, exposure to pesticides,   excessive alcohol and even a poor diet - encouraging your partner to increase his intake of phytonutrients can go a long way in helping to ensure you get pregnant!

The Super Fertility Nutrients: What To Eat Right Now!

While there are literally thousands of health-giving phytonutrients found in a variety of fruits, vegetables, nuts and grains, when it comes to boosting fertility most the most valuable compounds are grouped in three important categories.

They are: Phenolic Acids, Flavonoids and Carotinoids.

While each group contains a number of key individual phytonutrients that can boost fertility, for the most part they work as a team in a concept known as "Food Synergy". As you read earlier this is a nutritional concept that tells us that " the whole" can be greater can the sum of it's parts. And by that I mean that together these nutrients work in consort to provide your reproductive system with more help and more boosting power than when they are eaten on their own.

What follows is a quick rundown of some of their more outstanding fertility -boosting effects and how to choose the foods that can help you obtain them!

The Fertility PhytoNutrients:

GROUP # 1: PHENOLIC ACIDS

If you are like most women, exposure to environmental pollutants are hard to avoid. Whether it be too much sun, exposure to cigarette smoke, the chemicals in the environment, or even products you use in your home, it can be hard to live in today's world and not be affected.

But the good news is that natural compounds known as phenolic acids can offer you protection from all of these factors - and in the process help ensure your fertility as well.

In fact, one particular type of phenolic acid making huge headlines right now is "reservatrol". This is a natural compound that the plants manufacture in response to environmental stress. So, for example, when they are exposed to elements that might harm them - including things like air pollution and pesticides - they begin to manufacture more reservatrol.

So, it's not hard to see why this compound is so closely associated with overcoming the stressors of modern day living - particularly that which causes "oxidative stress" on cells.

But reservatrol is only one type phenolic acid - and there are numerous others found in a variety of fruits and vegetables. Working synergistically, they work to protect your heart and blood vessels, which is key to ensuring good blood flow to your ovaries and your uterus. And that can be key to a healthy conception.

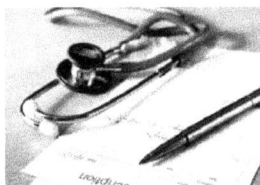

YOUR FERTILITY
FOOD PRESCRIPTION

Foods High In

Phenolic Acids

- Eat grapes, raspberries, strawberries, pomegranates & cranberries at least 3 to 5 times a week.

- At least once daily eat a citrus fruit, particularly red grapefruit. You can also choose oranges, lemons, limes or pink grapefruit.

- In moderation (if you are not actively trying to get pregnant) drink one glass of wine daily made from red grapes.

- Eat a handful of walnuts or pecans 3 times a week.

To Get Pregnant Faster ... Take a Deep Breath & Relax!

Studies show that some of the most common stress reduction techniques - such as meditation or yoga - can also have a beneficial effect on fertility. They work to calm stress hormones that can otherwise disrupt the menstrual cycle and keep you from conceiving.

A quick relaxation technique:

Put your hands on your tummy and breathe in, count to 5 and exhale. Do it 5 times several times a day - you won't believe the stress reduction in just a few days!

The Fertility PhytoNutrients:

GROUP # 2 : FLAVONOIDS

Flavonoids are a unique group of nutrients with many varied functions. Indeed, studies show they can have a direct impact on blood pressure, and they give added support to the heart by helping to maintain circulation in the smaller capillaries. And herein lies their first secret role in protecting fertility!

Indeed, your ovaries and the eggs inside them are literally "fed" by the tiniest capillaries - which bring fresh, oxygen-rich blood to these cells. When that circulation is compromised - and when your ovaries can't get the blood supply they need to thrive - studies show that egg production can dramatically falter.

One specific type of flavonoid   known as quercertin (found in grapes and cherries) also works on blood vessels, helping to keep tiny particles found naturally in your blood from sticking together and forming clumps. This function is key to helping you avoid miscarriage.

Still another type of flavonoid group are known as catechins. They're found in green tea and pack a mighty punch against cancers of the reproductive system, as well as protecting you from heart disease.

But it is really the impact of two more specific flavonoids - compounds known as anthocyanin and proantho cyanidins that actually help your fertility the most. Found in great abundance in fruits like blueberries and blackberries, they work to reduce the production of cytokines. These are inflammatory chemicals produced by various cells in the body, but particularly by fat cells.

In fact, the more fat cells your body has, the more cytokines you produce – so the more of these flavonoid compounds you need to counteract the damage. In terms of your fertility, studies show that inflammatory compounds can exert subtle negative effects on everything from egg production and ovulation, to egg transport inside your fallopian tube, to creating a hostile environment for sperm.

This is one reason why being overweight can make it harder to become pregnant.

In addition, these same inflammatory compounds can also play a role in insulin resistance and PCOS, as well as the menstrual related fertility disorder endometriosis. As such, if you suffer with any of these conditions then it's imperative that your diet contain foods high in these two important compounds.

Finally, there is still one more group of flavonoids you should know about. They fall under the heading of "isoflavones" Found in high concentrations in foods containing soy and peanuts, their link to fertility can be found in their natural estrogenic effects, which can be helpful in overcoming certain hormonal imbalances. They can also be important in conditions such as PCOS where estrogen production is abnormally low.

At the same time, however, I must caution you again about estrogenic plants. Indeed, if your estrogen levels are normal, eating too many foods high in isoflavones can have a negative effect on your fertility, so eat them only in moderation.

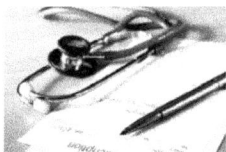

YOUR FERTILITY FOOD PRESCRIPTION

Foods High In

Flavonoids

Gain the fertility boosting effects of anthrocyanin and proantho cyanidins by adding more blue-red fruits to your diet including blueberries, raspberries, strawberries, ligonberries, cherries, currants, pomegranates, grapes and cranberries.

There is some good evidence to show t hat in moderation the flavonoids found in green tea can also be helpful - it contains 3 times the flavonoid content of black tea!

Flavonoids can also be found in grapes, cocoa, lentils, peaches and nectarines.

You can increase your intake of quercertin by eating more red grapes, cherries, kale, lettuce, apples, pears, nectarines, peaches, broccoli and onions, as well as drinking more tea.

The Fertility Phyto Nutrients:

GROUP # 3: CAROTINOIDS

Carotinoids are a family of nutrients containing many different compounds, the best known of which is beta carotene. Carotinoids are found in brightly colored fruits and vegetables such as carrots, mangoes, cantaloupe, sweet potatoes, tomatoes and watermelon.

As a powerful source of antioxidants, carotinoids offer protection from a wide range of diseases, from Alzheimer's to cancer.

But from a fertility standpoint these phytonutrients - which include compounds such as lycopene, lutein and zeaxanthin - are among the most important to include in your diet. Why?

First, carotinoids are what your body uses to make Vitamin A - a nutrient that is essential for the healthy growth and development of an embryo. In fact, when a serious Vitamin A deficiency exists, it's almost impossible to create a healthy embryo.

Moreover, research published by the European Society of Human Reproduction and Embryology also demonstrated how carotinoids are essential to the development of healthy follicular fluid – the semi-liquid substance which surrounds your egg and aids in growth and fertilization. Because follicular fluid appears to get it's supply of beta carotine from the bloodstream, it stands to reason that when levels are low, eggs may not get what they need to develop properly, and fertilize quickly and easily.

Also important are animal studies showing that beta carotene impacts brain chemicals necessary for the release of your egg. In fact some studies show that without adequate beta carotene, ovulation can't occur.

Moreover, a healthy corpus luteum (the shell your ovulated egg leaves behind) is naturally rich in beta carotene. Since this is one of the major sources of progesterone - a hormone that helps prepare your uterus for a healthy conception - fortifying your corpus luteum with additional beta carotene may help optimize your chances for a healthy implantation.

When it comes to your partner's fertility, beta carotene plays an equally important role. Indeed, a carotinoid compound known as "lycopene" has been shown to be necessary for the production of quality sperm.

So, to help you get pregnant even faster, you should make certain your partner pays special attention to foods containing this nutrient. The most potent sources include cooked tomatoes, so make sure he fills up on pizza with extra sauce, or puts plenty of ketchup on his burger. Tomato juice and baked tomatoes also contain lycopene.

> *Top your pizza with lots of cooked tomatoes and other veggies & it becomes a super fertility food for you & your partner! !*

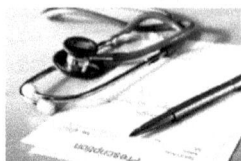

YOUR FERTILITY FOOD PRESCRIPTION

Foods High In

Carotinoids

- At least three times a week eat carrots, butternut squash, tomatoes, sweet potatoes, cantaloupe, kale or mangoes.

- To add more lycopene to your diet eat more tomatoes, watermelon, guava, plus red and white grapefruit.

- To maximize levels of lutein eat more avocados, oranges, and leafy green vegetables.

- For more beta carotene, try adding more apricots, papayas, plantains, broccoli, celery, pumpkin, spinach and winter squash to your diet.

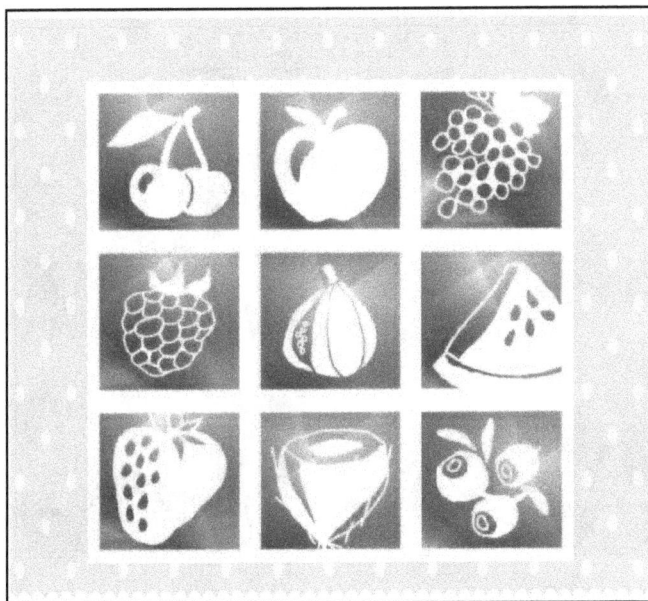

The Colors of Fertility

Taking advantage of all the important phytonutrients found in fruits and vegetables is easier than you think!

In fact, all you need do is add more colorful foods to your plate every day! Indeed, studies show that many of the most important phytonutrients identified to date are the same compounds that give fruits and vegetables their vivid, natural colors.

So the more "colors" you have on your plate, the more likely it is that you will be receiving a good variety of powerful, fertility-boosting phytonutrients.

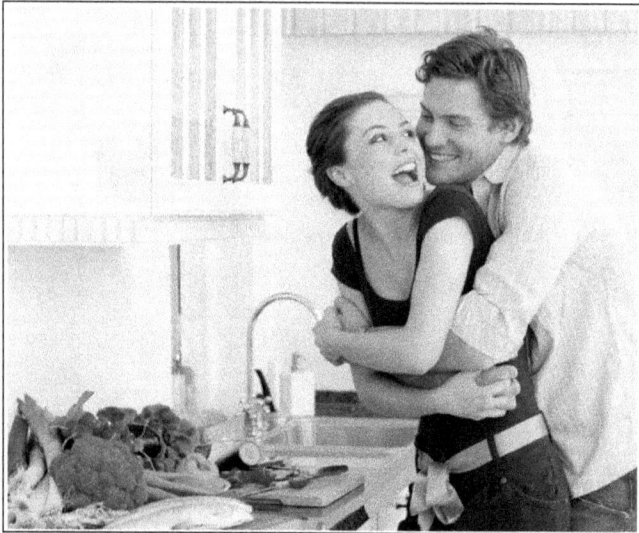

To Get Pregnant Faster - Stop & Smell The Produce!

Did you know that simply smelling fruits and vegetables might help you get pregnant? It's true!

A new study published in the journal of Agricultural and Food Chemistry found that many fruits and vegetables contain an aromatic compound known as linalool.

Inhaling the scent, say scientists causes a measurable reduction in stress hormones such as cortisol. It also helps calm down over 100 genes that go into overdrive as a result of the stress response.

Since there is good evidence that reducing stress levels can increase fertility, the "scent of pregnancy" may very well be lingering in the produce section of your favorite supermarket!

CHAPTER SIX

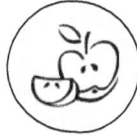

The Secret Is Out:
Fats Can Help You Get Pregnant Faster!

O nce upon a time - in the not too distant past - dietary fat was considered the number one health enemy.

In fact, you might already know that foods high in both fat and calories have been blamed for not only our burgeoning waistlines but also our increased risk of heart disease, high blood pressure, stroke - and some problems related to fertility.

That said, one of the more important facts to come to light in recent years is the idea that not all fats are alike. Much like carbohydrates, which are divided into two distinct subgroups, so too are fats.

So while some fats remain clearly harmful to your fertility - and you'll read more about those in a few moments - there are others which can actually make you more fertile - and help you get pregnant faster! And those are the ones I want to concentrate on right now!

The Good Fats That Help You Get Pregnant Fast!

When it comes to the "good" fertility fats, those at the very top of the list are known as MUFAs - short for mono-unsaturated fatty acids.

Derived from sources such as olives, nuts and fruits like avocados, these fats help the body to function more healthfully, including decreasing some of the effects of "bad fats", such as reducing cholesterol.

In addition, when paired with the fertility phytonutrients found in fruits and vegetables, these "healthy fats" work even better, stabilizing blood sugar levels and normalizing hormones necessary for optimum fertility.

Moreover, there is good evidence to show that a diet which replaces saturated fats with mono-unsaturated fats can not only help you lose weight, but more importantly may also help decrease inflammation associated with fertility robbing conditions such as endometriosis and PCOS. A little later in this book you'll learn more about how inflammation can impact every woman's fertility.

But MUFAs are not alone on the healthy pantry shelf. Right along side them are another group of fats known as PUFAs - short for polyunsaturated fatty acids.

Among this group are compounds known as "essential fatty acids" or EFAs, which directly impact the production of hormone-like compounds that not only regulate blood pressure, blood clotting and blood fats, but also insulin production. In terms of your fertility, however, two specific EFAs play a critical role. They are Omega 3 and Omega 6. And what's important about these two nutrients is that while they are essential to your health and your fertility, they are the only two EFAs your body cannot make on it's own. You must, in fact, get them from either foods or supplements.

Omega 3: The Super Sonic Fertility Booster!

While both Omega 3 and Omega 6 are important, when it comes to boosting fertility, it is Omega 3 fatty acids that hold the most significance. In particular it is two specific Omega 3 fatty acids - compounds known as eicosapentaenic acid (EPA) and docosahexanoic acid (DHA) - that can make the biggest dietary difference in how quickly you get pregnant.

Found in foods such as cold water fish, flax seeds and walnuts, these compounds appear to have a direct impact on ovulation, as well as working hard to protect you from the fertility robbing effects of both a high carbohydrate diet and in particular, insulin resistance.

While this is important for all women, it is particularly vital if you have been diagnosed with PCOS. Indeed, in one study published in the Journal of Clinical Endocrinology and Metabolism in 2004, researchers found that simply adding more of these Omega 3 fatty acids to the daily diet had enough of an impact on hormone production to kick-start ovulation in women with PCOS.

> Fish is one of the most plentiful sources of Omega 3 fatty acids but this important fertility nutrient can also be found in flax seeds, walnuts and many fortified foods!

Other research has shown that these same essential fatty acids can have a powerful anti-inflammatory effect on endometriosis, and in the process help reverse many of it's fertility-robbing effects as well.

But it's not just women with these specific conditions who can benefit from these powerful, natural compounds. Indeed studies show that these two Omega 3 fatty acids can encourage conception in every woman by reducing inflammation caused by, among other things, a poor diet. In doing so they also help counter the fertility-robbing effects of a number of types of hormone imbalances.

Moreover, these same compounds can also help increase blood flow to the uterus, which in turn can help insure a healthy implantation thus reducing the risk of miscarriage. Once you are pregnant, these same two omega 3 fatty acids can help promote the growth of your baby, mostly by increasing blood flow to the placenta - the sac that protects and nourishes the embryo in your womb.

Eating foods high in omega 3 fatty acids before you get pregnant may help you conceive a smarter baby!

Moreover, a diet rich in omega 3 fatty acids both before and after you get pregnant can reduce your risk of premature birth, help you avoid pre-eclampsia, (a dangerous rise in blood pressure that can occur during pregnancy) and reduce your risk of gestational diabetes. After you give birth these same two nutrients can decrease your risk of post partum depression!

And if that were not enough to convince you to add these nutrients to your diet, studies show that moms who consume lots of heart-healthy omega 3 fatty acids may give birth to a smarter baby - with all indications this nutrient contributes to brain development in the womb and the development of superior intelligence later in life!

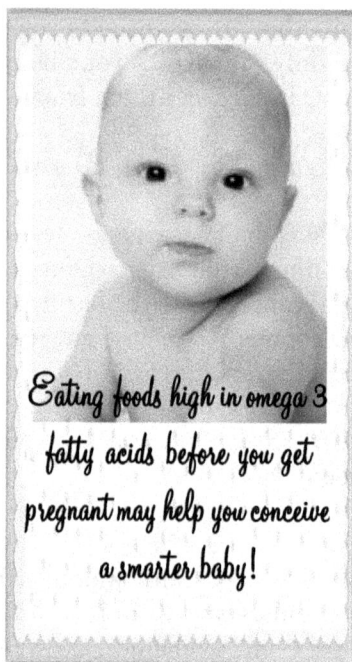

Keep The Balance & Get Pregnant Fast!

But there is still one more important reason to make sure you include enough omega-3 fatty acids in your daily diet: You need them to balance the impact of the much more plentiful omega-6 fatty acids, which are plentiful in soybean oil, cotton seed oil and corn oil, used in preparation of so many foods.

Indeed, as good as omega 6 fatty acids can be in terms of helping to reduce inflammation, when they are not balanced with sufficient amounts of omega-3s they can actually become a source of inflammation in your body. When this occurs it not only interferes with both your fertility and with a healthy pregnancy, it also increases your risk of diabetes and heart disease.

Moreover, when your intake of omega 6 rises too high – with no balance from omega 3's - it promotes the formation of blood clots, increasing your risk of heart attack and stroke, as well as miscarriage. In fact I have seen a number of patients who were able to overcome chronic miscarriage simply by balancing their intake of omega 3 and omega 6 fatty acids.

The very latest research shows that the most promising health effects of essential fatty acids overall are achieved through a proper balance of omega-3s and omega-6s. The ratio to shoot for is roughly 4 parts omega-3s to 1 part omega- 6s.

While this may sound like it involves some complicated mathematics, it's really just a matter of eating a healthy, balanced diet - one that includes varied sources of both omega 3 and omega 6.

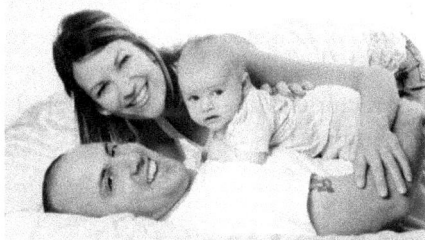

Today, many products, including yogurt, soy milk, eggs, egg whites, some brands of cereal and whole wheat bread are fortified with DHA. Read the labels to know for sure!

One Final Caution: Know Your Omega 3's

While loading up your diet with foods rich in omega 3 fatty acids in one way to help insure your fertility, finding the right sources is also important.

Certainly, fish remains the most potent and complete source of omega 3 fatty acids you can find. But if you have concerns about mercury, or if you simply aren't in love with fish, there are other foods that also contain this nutrient, including walnuts, flax seed oil, and some brands of mayonnaise.

That said, when it comes to boosting your fertility, nutritionist Elizabeth Somer, RD says that relying on these foods alone could still mean you come up nutritionally short. Why?

"What you get in foods like walnuts and flax seed oil is an omega-3 acid known as ALA - alpha-linoleic acid," says Somer.

While it's good for your health she says, in order to gain the full benefits of omega 3 these foods require that your body convert ALA to DHA - the kind of omega 3 most helpful to fertility. But the problem with the conversion, says Somer, is that a variety of individual health factors - including your overall nutritional status- can sometimes hamper that process. So, you end up with less protection than you realize.

The solution: There are a variety of foods now available that are fortified with DHA so no conversion process is necessary! These include certain brands of eggs, egg whites, soy milk, some brands of whole wheat bread and some breakfast cereals, and incorporating them into your diet can be very helpful. To make sure you're getting foods that are fortified, check the label and sure it says "Fortified with DHA".

Also remember, for some extra "fertility insurance" you can take omega-3 supplements, alone or in conjunction with foods high in omega-3. This will help ensure you are getting enough of this very vital compound.

The Fats That Harm Fertility: What To Avoid

As you just read, there are certainly types of dietary fat that can make a huge difference in helping you get pregnant fast. But while we were discovering all the good news about these "good fats", we also learned a great deal more about the impact of "bad fats" - and the foods that contain them.

Among those fats now considered to the most harmful to your general health, perhaps none is more threatening to your fertility than those known as "trans fats". These are man-made compounds that occur during conversion of liquid oil into a solid shortening. They are frequently used in many commercial baked goods and fast foods because they help extend the "shelf life" of foods.

The problem is that while these hybrid shortenings may extend the life of foods on the supermarket shelves, the trans fats that result do the opposite for those of us who consume them. Indeed, trans fats are now believed to be a direct link to heart disease, insulin resistance, type 2 diabetes, and now, infertility.

Indeed, in one study recently published in a leading nutrition journal researchers found that women whose diet include just 4 grams of trans fat per day had a whopping 93% increase in fertility problems related to ovulation.

But how, exactly, do trans fats harm your chances of getting pregnant?

While no one knows for certain, many believe they incite inflammatory reactions within the body - a condition that not only impacts ovulation, but may even affect the health of your fallopian tubes. Trans fats also impact the way sugar is metabolized, so, much like quick-burn "simple" carbohydrates, they play a role in exacerbating insulin sensitivity. As you read earlier, this can impact ovarian function, particularly egg production and release.

Eat well before you get pregnant & you will give birth to a healthier baby! Not surprisingly the same foods that are good for Mom are great for baby!

Moreover, my personal research and experience has shown that the inflammation related to trans fats also impacts endometriosis, oftentimes making symptoms and the associated fertility problems much worse.

The good news: By simply reducing your consumption of foods high in trans fat you can not only improve endometriosis symptoms, but also increase your chance of getting pregnant.

An Important Caution ...

If you take the time to read food and nutrition labels you can avoid trans fats and still eat many of your favorite snacks & treats! Remember however, that many foods which say they contain No Trans Fat can legally contain up to .5 grams - which can really add up at the end of the day!

And this is true both for women who have this disorder and those who do not.

And now I'm happy to report that avoiding trans fats is easier than ever, thanks to some major changes within the food industry, with many companies making a real effort to remove these fats from their products.

In Denmark, where I grew up, the impact of dietary fat has always been a major health concern, which is why I wasn't at all surprised to learn in 2003 that they became the first nation in the world to ban trans fats from all commercial food products. Today many countries and major cities around the world have followed suit.

Indeed, in many parts of the US and Europe, trans fats are now banned from use by restaurants, particularly fast food places, which were the biggest offenders. As a result, companies such as

KFC, Taco Bell, Wendy's, Chili's and Starbucks have all announced efforts to eliminate or drastically reduce trans fats in their products.

Moreover , thanks to new FDA guidelines, there are now fewer trans fats lurking in popular foods on supermarket shelves - and if you read food labels it's easy to tell which companies are making the effort to cut the fat!

So, if you're trying to get pregnant, spending a little time doing some "supermarket reading" could benefit your fertility in myriad ways.

That said, it's also important to point out that while many snack and fast foods boast they contain "NO TRANS FAT", legally that means they can still contain up to .5 grams or one-half gram of trans fat per serving.

Since we all know that serving sizes are deceiving (studies show most of us automatically double the suggested serving size), it's easy to see how you can consume 4 grams or more of trans fat a day and still think you aren't getting any!

Add to this the foods that you know contain trans fats and you eat them anyway - like donuts or French fries - and it's even easier to reach or surpass that 4 gram -a-day mark that studies show can interrupt fertility.

To keep this from happening try to reduce or cut out all sources that you know of , and when you can't cut it out, eat as little as possible of those foods. At the same time, loading up on fruits and veggies will not only leave less room for foods high in trans fats it can also help counter some of the fertility-robbing effects of the trans fats you do consume.

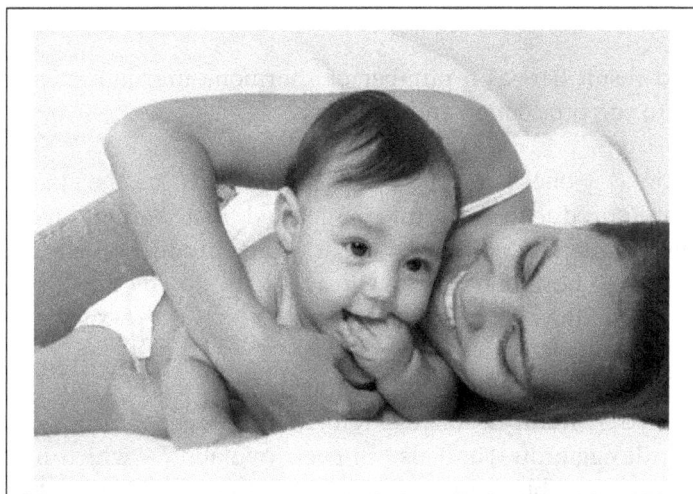

Reduce This One Fat ...& Watch Fertility Soar!

While avoiding trans fats is one way to get pregnant faster, studies also show that avoiding saturated fats is another way to boost your fertility. These are the mostly animal-based fats that come primarily from sources like red meat, processed foods, poultry skin and egg yolks.

How can avoiding saturated fat help you get pregnant faster?

Much like trans fat, saturated fats increase insulin resistance, making it much harder for your body to clear sugar from your blood. But more than that, saturated fats can also increase the production of triglycerides, a byproduct of saturated fat that is stored in our cells after we eat that big juicy steak or steamy hamburger and fries.

Besides increasing your risk of heart attack and stroke, triglycerides can also impact your pancreas, which is the organ that actually produces insulin. When your pancreas cells are affected, insulin production becomes erratic, and sugars can't be cleared as effectively from blood.

The end result here is a number of hormone imbalances, some related to egg production and release.

Indeed, in one recent study published in the journal Human Reproduction, doctors suggested that a diet high in saturated fats can directly impact the production of key reproductive hormones as well as slow down the overall functioning of the ovaries.

There is also some evidence to show that these "bad fats" can reduce your number of egg follicles (the "seeds" from which your fertile egg grows) and also impact ovulation – which is the major stumbling block to getting pregnant for a vast majority of women.

Saturated Fats, Pregnancy & Fertility Treatments

Of even greater concern : If you do manage to get pregnant while consuming a lot of these nasty fats, your risk of gestational diabetes also increases. Continue to eat these foods after your baby is born and you could see a decrease in the quality of your breast milk - and that may impact your baby's brain development.

Moreover, some very new and interesting research also published in the journal Human Reproduction suggests that even if you do manage to make and ovulate an egg, a diet high in saturated fat could prevent that egg from being fertilized. And this may be true even if you're undergoing sophisticated fertility treatments such as IVF (in vitro fertilization). Indeed, in this same study doctors examined eggs that failed to fertilize in women who were having IVF and found that the majority of them contained high levels of saturated fats.

The good news however is that by replacing the "bad fats" in your diet with some of the "good fats" we talked about earlier, you can have your cake and eat it too - or at least some of it!

How Ice Cream Can Help You Get Pregnant Faster!

If you've even been on a weight loss diet – or even thought about losing weight –then you know the importance of avoiding high fat dairy products . Indeed, items like whole milk, ice cream or full fat yogurt can really pack on the pounds!

Moreover, as you just read, high fat dairy foods are also high in saturated animal fat , which you now know can cause inflammatory reactions within the body that, for the most part, are bad for fertility.

That's one reason why researchers were so surprised to discover what I like to refer to as "The Ice Cream Paradox" - powerful new research indicating that certain high fat dairy products, but particularly ice cream and whole milk – may be the one exception to the saturated fat "rule".

Indeed, when consumed in moderate amounts these foods appear to encourage rather than discourage a quick and easy conception. And that's precisely what a group of Harvard researchers found out when they reanalyzed data from the massive Nurses Health Study.

Here researchers learned that one or two daily servings of whole milk, as well as products made from whole milk such as ice cream and full fat yogurt, appear to have protective effects on ovulation. Ironically, the otherwise healthier skim and low fat milk products seemed to have the *opposite effect*.

Certainly, this contradicts not only common sense, but also current nutritional guidelines which tell us that foods high in animal fat are bad for our heart, blood pressure and yes, even our fertility.

At the same time, however, when you look a little deeper at the differences between high and low fat dairy products, the Harvard findings begin to make some sense.

More specifically, estrogen and other reproductive hormones are stored in fat – not only in humans, but also in animals, particularly cows. So when milk – or milk byproducts such as ice cream or cheese – are fully fatted, they contain an abundance of these hormones. But remove the fat from the milk – and the resulting milk products - and you no longer have these extra hormones.

In older, post menopausal women this reduction of hormone stimulation can be a good thing, since too much estrogen during these years can increase the risk of certain cancers.

Conversely, however, some researchers now believe that an abundance of estrogen in the childbearing years can be good for some women, particularly those who may already have ovulatory problems and as such are considered estrogen deficient

This includes women who are very thin, or particularly those who exercise a great deal, which can, in some instances, disrupt or reduce estrogen production.

In any event, when this is the case, then the extra estrogen found in full-fat dairy products may offer enough of a boost to tip the scales from fertile to infertile!

According to the Harvard findings, the high fat dairy products most likely to encourage conception included whole milk and ice cream. The foods most likely to have a negative impact on fertility included sherbet and frozen yogurt which appeared to contribute to ovulatory dysfunction - or at the very least did nothing to improve ovarian function.

What's more, the findings were also dose-responsive. The more low fat dairy products a woman ate, the more difficulty she appeared to have getting pregnant.

Conversely, the more full-fat dairy products she ate, the less likely she was to have a problem conceiving.

Certainly this research is still considered preliminary. Moreover, remember that it applies only to women who are not making enough estrogen on their own - particularly those who are underweight. And when you look at it in this perspective, the finding is not so unusual or even so new. In fact over 20 years ago I recommended in the first edition of my book Getting Pregnant:What You Need To Know Now that women who were underweight and had ovulatory problems should eat more ice cream and whole fat dairy products.

At the same time - then and now - I also suggested that if you are overweight you may actually be producing too much estrogen , leading to a hormone imbalance that can cause infertility. When this is the case, increasing your intake of whole milk and full fat ice cream could do you more harm than good.

Who Needs Ice Cream - Who Doesn't !

The bottom line: If you are not overweight and want to try high fat dairy products as a way to encourage fertility, then go ahead and give it try - just be sure to do so in moderation! Indeed, one serving per day of full fat milk and two half cup servings of full fat ice cream per week is all you need to gain

A Little Goes A Long Way!

In one Harvard University study, the more high fat dairy products a woman ate, the more fertile she was!

The more low-fat dairy products she ate, the more problems she had getting pregnant!

But remember, the amount of ice cream you need to improve fertility is only about ½ pint per week!

the benefits discussed in the Harvard study. More   importantly, if you do add these foods to your diet, be certain to compensate to some degree by reducing the amount of calories you get from other foods, and by reducing your intake of saturated fats from other source, such as red meat.   You should also reduce your intake of snack foods high in trans fat, such as potato chips, French fries or donuts. Doing so will help balance the extra calories and prevent you from gaining too much weight, which can hamper your fertility.

If you are already overweight, you can still try giving your fertility the ice cream boost, but limit your intake to no more than two servings per week - and skip the whole fat milk.

When you do get pregnant, all women should switch back to *low fat* dairy products. While it's important to include the nutrients from dairy foods during pregnancy, it's also important not to gain too much weight. So by switching over to low fat dairy you and your baby can gain all the health benefits without the risks!

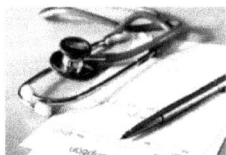

YOUR FERTILITY FOOD PRESCRIPTION:

Dietary Fat

Include as many of these foods as you
can in 3 to 5 meals a week.

*Salmon * Tuna * Mackerel
* Walnuts * Cashews * Pecans * Peanuts
* Flax Seed Oil * Olive Oil
*Canola Oil * Ground flax
* Granola.

You should try to limit, or when possible avoid the following foods which are high in saturated fats and triglycerides.

Fatty cuts of beef such as chuck.
Meat drippings or gravy made from drippings.
Bacon, sausage, and processed meats
The skin of duck, chicken or turkey.
Egg yolks & Butter
Fat or oil that is hard or in stick form
such as lard, shortening or margarine.
Hydrogenated vegetable oils.
Coconut, coconut oil, palm oil, and palm kernel oil.
Full fat cheeses, sour cream, cottage cheese.
Processed grain products such as cookies, and pastries.

Also be aware that depending on how they are cooked, many seemingly healthy "fast foods" - like fish sandwiches for example - could contain high levels of trans fat.

CHAPTER SEVEN

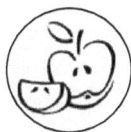

Six Super Fertility Food Boosters

The Super Fertility Food Prescription To Help You Get Pregnant Even Faster!

*W*ould you believe it if I told you that some of the most delicious foods, some of the most popular foods, some of the foods you probably already love are also among the most powerful fertility food boosters available?

It's true! From luscious fruits to snack foods, from the favorite toppings on your burgers to your favorite beverages, science has shown us that when it comes to getting pregnant fast, certain foods do have some "super powers".

And while all of the foods mentioned in this fertility food guide thus far can definitely help you get pregnant faster, the specific foods you will discover in this chapter are something very special.

I like to call them my **Super Secret   Fertility Foods** - super because research shows can make a huge difference in your ability to get pregnant - and secret because not many people are aware of their powers!

While most of these foods contain many of the same key phytonutrients discussed in a previous chapter, they also contain additional vitamins, nutrients or other factors that have been linked to both robust health and increased fertility. As such, adding them to your daily diet, even in small quantities, can go a long way in helping you to get pregnancy quickly and easily.

Remember, however, that the best   way   to   improve   your fertility is to improve your overall health - and that can only happen when your nutritional profile is balanced. So while you might be tempted to eat only the "super foods" mentioned here, I caution you not to do that.

Not only is it vital to your fertility to eat a balanced diet, the true boosting power of these "super foods" comes only when they are part of a nutritionally sound eating plan.

So, with this in mind, I invite you to dive in to the following chapter and get your food creativity going! I know you will find many new and exciting ways to incorporate these foods into your daily meal plans.

Also important: Most of the Super Foods listed in this chapter are also good for male fertility, so be sure to enlist your partner's help in the kitchen, then share your fertility-boosting meals together!

Remember ... foods that help your fertility can also help your partner's fertility!

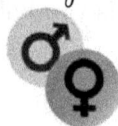

Super Fertility Food Booster # 1:

Organic Wild Blueberries

It's hard to pick up a magazine or open your lap top without seeing a news story about the powerful, health-giving benefits of blueberries!

As you read earlier, these tiny fruits are packed with a powerful phytonutrient known as anthocyanins - a natural compound that is responsible for giving blueberries their deep, rich color. But it also does much more than that.

This powerful natural chemical reduces the impact of inflammation body-wide, and in doing so benefits nearly every segment of reproduction. This includes making and ovulating healthy eggs, helping sperm and egg meet, keeping your fallopian tubes clear for the easy transport of your embryo to your uterus, and finally, keeping the lining of your uterus healthy so that your implantation and your pregnancy can be healthy and strong.

And if that were not enough, studies show that adding just a half cup of blueberries to your daily diet can lower cholesterol, fight high blood pressure, reduce the risk of memory loss and brain motor function disorders, and even protect you from cancer!

While all blueberries are good for fertility, there are some that offer an exceptional boost. Indeed, there is now good evidence to show that berries which are grown organically may pack a significantly greater antioxidant punch than berries grown in the conventional way. And this means they might offer your fertility an ever bigger boost.

Moreover, scientists have also discovered that where blueberries are grown can also make a difference, particularly in regard to their nutritional value. Among the blueberries offering the biggest bang for your nutritional buck are those grown in the wilds of Alaska.

According to research conducted by National Institutes of Health scientist Maureen McKenzie, Ph.D, thanks to certain geo-adaptations the Alaskan blueberry is able to withstand even the harshest climates of the frozen tundra. Not coincidentally, these adaptations involved a dramatic increase in natural antioxidant production - up to 7 times that which is found in berries grown in warmer climates. And the best news of all: That super protection is passed on to all who eat these berries!

If you can't get your hands on Alaskan blueberries, there are supplements available - most notably Aurora Blue, made from pure Alaskan blueberries. Even with processing, they still maintain an ORAC score (the measure of a product's antioxidant content) four times that found in wild Maine blueberries and seven times that grown in other locations.

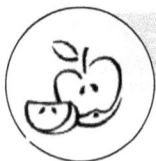

To satisfy your sweet tooth and boost your fertility at the same time, try blueberry jam! One brand in particular - Crofters - combines organic blueberries with natural sugar & other organic fruits to offer a super high anti -oxidant jam that is also delicious!

Super Fertility Food Booster # 2:

Cruciferous Vegetables!

While all vegetables have some capacity to enhance your fertility, if you want to get pregnant faster and easier munch on some broccoli, cauliflower, Brussels sprouts, kale, cabbage, and bok choy. How can they help you? .

As an interrelated group known as "cruciferous vegetables" these mostly green veggies are packed with fertility-enhancing phytochemicals, vitamins, minerals and fiber - all compounds that not only protect your fertility and your heart, but also act as powerful cancer-fighting warriors.

In one study funded by the National Cancer Institute, researchers found that body-wide oxidative cell stress (including that which adversely impacts fertility) dropped by 22% after just a few weeks of a diet high in cruciferous vegetables. Now if you think you can get the same effects by popping a vitamin supplement, guess again. The study also showed that those who took a vitamin supplement instead of eating the veggies saw almost no decrease in oxidative stress.

But this isn't the only way in which these veggies can help your fertility!

Cruciferous veggies like broccoli, cauliflower and cabbage are not only good for your fertility they can also help your partner too! So remember to encourage him to eat healthy and fill his plate with tons of sperm-loving veggies!

Indeed, studies have shown that natural compounds found in these veggies may promote healthy estrogen metabolism - a hormone which is essential for every stage of reproduction, from egg development to maturation, from ovulation to implantation.

But the news gets even better! These veggies are not only healthy, they're smart! And here's why: There are two pathways through which your body metabolizes estrogen. One way results in a healthy metabolic by-product known as 2-hydroxyestrone. The other way results in a more toxic by-product, a chemical known as 16 alphahydroxyestrone. In fact studies show that women who metabolize estrogen through this pathway are much more susceptible to breast cancer and possibly, some forms of infertility.

So how do veggies make a difference?

The natural compounds found in these vegetables - particularly two natural chemicals known as 13C and DIM , appear to shift the pathway through which estrogen is metabolized, encouraging production of the more healthy metabolites and lowering production of the more toxic ones. This not only reduces the risk of breast but also cervical cancer in women.

And while the research linking these compounds to fertility is still in it's early stages, I and many of my European colleagues believe that when you combine the powerful antioxidant protection these vegetables provide with the positive healthful changes in estrogen metabolism, it translates into healthier and better quality eggs overall. And that means getting pregnant will be faster and easier.

While three to four half-cup servings per day can offer optimal protection, even one to two servings per day can offer you important benefits. And remember, you can begin to see a difference in as little as two weeks!

" When you combine the powerful antioxidant protection of these vegetables with the positive healthful changes in estrogen metabolism it translates into healthier eggs overall... and that means you get pregnant faster & easier! "

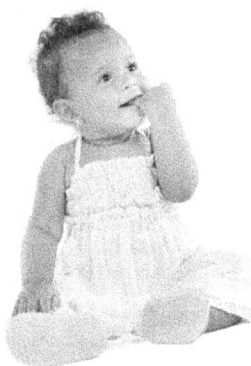

Super Fertility Food Booster # 3:
Onions & Garlic

When I was in medical school, the running joke in the gynecology department was that onions and garlic were the most effective method of birth control - because if you ate them every day no one would want to get close enough to get to know you!

But the truth is, these two powerful foods may , in fact, have the opposite effect – because at least on a biochemical level, they contain compounds that might just help you get pregnant!

Both onions and garlic are considered vegetable "cousins", belonging to the family of phytonutrients known as the "allylic sulfur compounds". Also part of the family are leeks, scallions and chives, and several other "bulb" vegetables.

But when it comes to your fertility, research shows it is onions and garlic, either alone or especially together, that appear to pack the biggest punch! What can they do for you?

First, research shows that compounds found in these vegetables are potent anti-cancer fighters, helping to protect against colon, stomach, breast and in particular ovarian cancer. In fact, studies show that even adding these vegetables to the diet after cancer has been diagnosed can help slow the growth of some of malignant tumors

But in terms of your fertility onions and garlic can play a key role in helping to repair damage to DNA, as well as regulating the life cycle of a cell. And that can have a powerful impact on getting pregnant. Why?

One of the ways in which fertility becomes impaired is via exposure to environmental toxins and pollutants - factors which ultimately break down cell walls and alter DNA. Thus, it stands to reason that any natural compounds which can halt this activity can also encourage fertility.

But the protection doesn't stop here. In a study published in the Journal of Nutrition in 2003 researchers found that extracts made from garlic powder also have a potent effect on cytokines - which as you just read earlier are the inflammatory chemicals that can impact fertility on many levels, particularly in those women diagnosed with endometriosis or PCOS.

Although it's not known for its "romantic" qualities, garlic contains many fertility-boosting nutrients - and not just for women! Because it's high in selenium - a key mineral for the production of healthy sperm - it's also considered to be a male fertility booster!

My suggestion is to include onions and garlic in at least one meal every day - but you don't have to eat a lot to get a lot of protection. Indeed, using them as a garnish on a salads, or mixing them in with other vegetables can add flavor to your meals while protecting your fertility. To sweeten your breath after eating these veggies try chewing on a sprig of parsley or watercress.

SIX SUPER FERTILITY FOOD BOOSTERS96

Super Fertility Food Booster # 4:
Green Tea

Although the facts surrounding the impact of green tea on fertility are still considered a bit controversial, increasingly research is showing that it can have a favorable impact on getting pregnant. One reason of course, is it's powerful antioxidant activity. Indeed, tea of any type is high in a phytonutrient known as polyphenols, a type of "flavonoid" with robust antioxidant activity.

But the polyphenols found in green tea are present in amounts as much as 3 times greater than that found in black tea – meaning it's antioxidant power is greater as well. And many experts now believe that this power can be a defining factor in those seeking to get pregnant.

A second chemical found in tea – a natural compound known as hypoxithine – is, oddly enough, the same chemical found in the follicular fluid that surrounds the eggs in your ovary. It works to help foster growth , development and eventually ovulation. Researchers theorize that the hypoxithine found in tea may have beneficial effects on egg production and growth as well.

Indeed, in one now-classic study published nearly a decade ago, researchers from Kaiser Permanente Health System found that women who drank as little as one-half cup of green tea daily nearly doubled their chances of conceiving! The same effect was not seen with other caffeinated beverages.

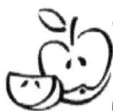

> *In one recent European study researchers found that a compound in green tea increased pregnancy rates significantly when used in conjunction with IVF by increasing the number of eggs available for fertilization!*

More recently a Stanford University study of 30 women, aged 24 to 46 who had not been able to conceive for up to three years, researchers found that a supplement containing green tea and several of the herbs and vitamins improved conception odds considerably. Indeed, one-third of the women taking the supplement were able to get pregnant within five months, compared to no pregnancies in the control group. While the researchers say they can't be certain if the effects were due to the green tea specifically, a new European animal study indicates it just might be the active component.

In this study, published in April 2008, researchers from the University of Bologna reported that when used in conjunction with IVF, a compound in green tea known as EGCG increased pregnancy rates significantly, mostly by increasing the number of eggs available for fertilization. Interestingly, however, when concentrations of EGCG were increased, the percentage of eggs actually went down.

What does this mean for you? As with most factors that impact our health, moderation is the key! While it seems clear that green tea can have beneficial effects on fertility, overdoing it may not be a good thing.

My suggestion: Drink up to 7 cups of green tea per week. This will likely bring you many health benefits including improving your fertility profile. That said, until we have more information on any potential problems, I would limit the amount to just 7 cups a week.

Super Fertility Food Booster # 5:

Almonds, Cashews, Walnuts & More!

Although foods that are high in fat are generally not good for your health or your fertility, that tenet changes dramatically when it comes to nuts. Indeed, there are almost 300 different types of nuts , and while they are high in fat (and calories) it's the type of fat they contain that makes them a healthy choice – and even a super fertility food.

How can they help you?

Nuts contain mostly mono-unsaturated and polyunsaturated oils – which, as you read earlier, are part of the family of "good fats" that can help lower cholesterol and have anti-inflammatory effects on your cells. Many nuts, but walnuts in particular, are also a good source of healthy omega-3 fatty acids – which can help build a stronger cell membrane and offer protection from free radical attack. For those of you who may be dealing with inflammatory conditions that impact fertility – such as endometriosis and PCOS – the healthy fats found in nuts can make a huge difference in not only your symptoms, but also in helping you conceive.

And if you love almonds – well you are in luck! Not only do they contain healthy fats, they are also one of the richest sources of antioxidants! According to researchers from Tufts University, after testing the skins and kernels of eight varieties of California almonds, they found the phytonutrients contained in these nuts offered the highest level of free radical damage protection of any flavonoid group!

In fact, ounce for ounce when you eat almonds you're getting the same level of phytonutrient protection found in broccoli, black and green tea, and red onions!

In addition, nuts, as well as seeds are high in a natural compound known as "phytosterols" - a plant based fat that recently gained lots of attention for it's ability to lower cholesterol. You've probably already heard of the term "sterols" in regard to "healthy" margarines such as Benecol or Smart Balance.

But what you might not know is that a recent analysis of 27 different varieties of nuts as well as certain seeds (see Super Fertility Booster # 6) found that these foods had among the highest concentration of healthy sterols.

And here's the really big surprise: In addition to reducing cholesterol these same plant sterols also help decrease the risk of some cancers as well as enhancing the immune system - and therein lies another very quiet but very powerful link to fertility. What is it?

First, when your immune system is strong your body is better able to defend itself against the ravages of a number of fertility-robbing infections. But that's just the beginning of the protection. Indeed, in a now-classic study conducted at the Mount Sinai School of Medicine by my colleague, fertility expert Dr. Norbert Gleicher, a weakened immune system may be to blame for a number of different types of infertility.

In his research, women who were prone to fertility problems had a significantly higher level of autoimmune antibodies, not only in their blood, but also in the fluid that surrounds a fertilized egg.

In fact, in one study , Dr. Gleicher found that women with abnormal levels of autoimmune antibodies who underwent IVF, had a pregnancy rate of just one-fifth that of women with normal antibody levels. So, it's easy to see why nuts, and the immune system protection they offer, can be a powerful fertility food.

Also important to remember: Nuts are a good source of protein, which as you read earlier in the book, is key to healthy ovulation and egg production. However, unlike red meat and other animal sources of protein, that which is found in nuts is healthier overall, for your heart and for your fertility.

Lastly, nuts are also a potent source of fiber, which means they can help balance blood sugar and reduce the risk of insulin resistance and in doing so help keep ovulation on track.

Of course nuts are also high in calories, so you don't want to over do it ! In fact, just a small handful of mixed nuts per day is more than enough to give your fertility a boost! Plus, if you eat them instead of chips or cookies, you'll keep your calorie intake balance and do a good deed for your body and your fertility!

As healthy as nuts can be, there is, however, one precaution to heed. Some nuts, but particularly peanuts, are high in the phytonutrient isoflavones. Which means that, much like soy, they can also be a significant source of plant estrogens.

If your estrogen levels are dwindling or low - if you are past age 35 , for example, or if you have PCOS - then peanuts can give you an estrogen boost that might help you get pregnant.

At the same time, however, if your estrogen levels are already high in relation to progesterone (one tell-tale sign would be raging PMS before every menstrual cycle) then the plant estrogens in some nuts might tip your fertility balance in the wrong direction.

While eating a small handful of peanuts a day probably won't "rock your estrogen boat", if you do find that eating these nuts increases your symptoms of PMS, then you should definitely cut down on the amount you eat, or mix them with other nuts such as walnuts, cashews or pistachios.

Moreover, if you are overweight, you should also consider limiting your peanut consumption. First, because of the high calories, but more importantly because of the estrogen connection. As you read earlier, the more fat cells you have the more estrogen your body produces, so you don't need the extra stimulation these nuts can provide.

Beer, Peanuts & Fertility

If your partner likes to wind down the night with a glass of beer and handful of nuts ..think twice if having a baby is in your immediate plans! Both beer and peanuts contain enough plant estrogens to slow down sperm production and motility - and make getting pregnant harder!

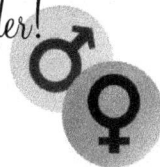

Super Fertility Food Booster #6 : Sunflower Seeds, Pumpkin Seeds & Wheat Germ!

When I was a small boy growing up in Denmark, my mother frequently fed my brother, my sister and I snacks made with both wheat germ and a variety of different seeds.

At the time we all wanted more cookies and pies – but in a classic case of " Mother Knows Best", I now know that Mom had our best health interests at heart! Indeed, adding foods like wheat germ, plus sunflower, pumpkin and sesame seeds to your diet can not only protect you from both cancer and heart disease, it might just increase your fertility as well.

How? First these foods are a powerful source of plant sterols, which as you just read can impact your immunity and ultimately your fertility.

But these seeds also contain relatively high concentrations of omega 3 fatty acids – which can boost fertility in a variety of ways, including stimulating the production of sex hormones in both men and women.

Sunflower seeds as well as pumpkin seeds work in harmony with fruits and vegetables to help boost your fertility and improve your overall health! Plus all you need is a handful 3 times a week to gain huge fertility benefits!

Moreover, pumpkin seeds, high in vitamin E and zinc, can be particularly beneficial for male fertility. Research shows that just ¼ to ½ cup a day can boost the overall health of a man's reproductive system and increase the concentration of healthier sperm overall.

If you are prone to miscarriage – or just want to ensure an extra healthy implantation, be sure to add more wheat germ to your diet. High in both vitamin E and selenium, research shows these two nutrients are essential to reducing the risk of pregnancy loss.

Wheat germ, as well as sunflower and sesame seeds are also high in vitamin B6, which is essential to not only produce female hormones, but to maintain proper ratios of estrogen and progesterone necessary for a quick and easy conception.

And finally, seeds, can also help provide much needed fiber in your diet. This can not only optimize your health overall, but also help reduce the risk of insulin resistance and all the fertility-robbing effects you read about earlier.

CHAPTER EIGHT

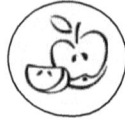

Beware

The Fertility Robbers!

Six Foods
You Need To Know More About!

When it comes to getting pregnant, fortunately there are almost no foods known to have an immediate, direct *harmful* effect on fertility.

So, in this respect, you never have to panic that you may have eaten the "wrong" food now, or in the past.

That said, there are a number of foods which can make it harder for you to get pregnant. While they may not have an immediate impact, over time, or when consumed in large quantities, they might make it more difficult for you to conceive.

I like to call these foods the "Fertility Robbers" - because if left unchecked they can literally "steal" your chances for a fast and healthy conception.

The good news: Not only can avoiding or eliminating these foods make a difference, when you replace them with healthy, fertility-promoting meals you also help counter damage that may have occurred - be it from a poor diet, the environment or a lifestyle issue such as smoking or being overweight.

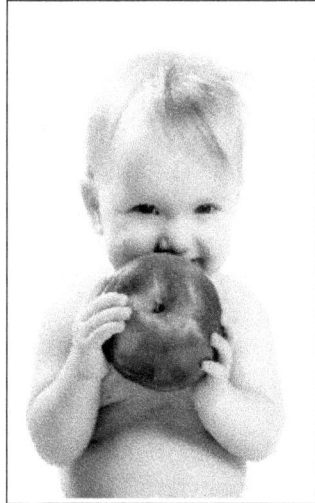

Certainly, some of these "robber foods" may be things you really enjoy - so it might be difficult to give them up completely. If this is the case, try to choose the one or two foods you just can't "live without" and eat them in moderation, while cutting out the others on the list.

Moreover, if you are eating a few foods that might not be the best choice for your fertility, try to counter the effects by making sure your diet includes at least a few of the "Super Fertility" foods you've already read about. Most important to include are the fruits and vegetables high in antioxidant protection.

Remember, the goal is to always strike a balance and then sit back and enjoy the choices you do make!

To help make choosing easier, what follows is important information you need to know about some of the most common "fertility food robbers" - including how and why they can interfere with your fertility.

If you choose wisely, you can still enjoy your most favorite foods without fear or worry and give your fertility a boost at the same time!

Fertility Robber #1:
Alcohol

While alcohol may not technically be considered a "food" - at least not in terms of nourishment - it certainly is part of our food culture.

For this reason and because it can have such a devastating effect on fertility, alcohol gets my vote as the number one item on your dinner table to avoid when you are trying to conceive.

You probably already know the dangers of drinking while you are pregnant - including a risk of fetal alcohol syndrome, a condition that can affect your baby's growth and development as well as their intelligence level, for life. Mothers who drink a great deal during pregnancy also subject their babies to growth problems, an increased risk of mental retardation, heart defects and an increased risk of a variety of serious health threats.

But in terms of fertility, drinking too much alcohol can actually keep you from getting pregnant. In one now classic British study of four hundred couples, even moderate drinking- as little as one glass of beer or wine a day - was found to decrease the chances for conception by a whopping 50 percent!

More recently studies have shown that regular use of alcohol can impact brain hormones necessary for ovulation. When consumption is high enough, ovulation can stop completely.

What's more heavy drinking may impact the lining of your uterus, keeping it from developing into the soft, spongy nest your embryo needs to implant and grow. In this way, heavy alcohol consumption may increase the risk of early miscarriage.

And it's not just *your* fertility that can be affected by alcohol - your partner's fertility can be affected as well. Indeed, studies show that even moderate alcohol intake can affect the health of sperm and keep it from fertilizing an egg.

Certainly, an occasional glass of wine or beer, or even an alcoholic drink now and again is not likely to do you or your partner any harm - particularly if you are young and healthy. Still, if you are trying to conceive and particularly if you are having problems getting pregnant quickly, it's a very good idea to cut out all alcohol for at least two months. Doing so will help to optimize your hormone production as well as increase egg production and release, which can help ensure a quicker and easier conception.

Cigarettes & Alcohol: A Bad Fertility Combo

For many women, alcohol goes hand in hand with a cigarette. And while I do recommend that you quit smoking when trying to conceive, if you can't stop smoking then don't combine cigarettes with alcohol. Studies show that when used together, they enhance the harmful effects of each other and do more damage to your fertility.

Fertility Robber # 2: Caffeine

If you're like many of my former patients you just can't start your day without a steaming cup of java jolt! In fact, when asked what food they could never give up, most of my patients always said "Coffee" without a moment's hesitation.

The problem, of course is that coffee – or more precisely its caffeine content - might be harmful to fertility. Though research is far from conclusive, there certainly are enough studies to make those of us in the fertility community sit up and take notice.

Among the most important is research conducted by Yale University on some 2,000 women. Here doctors found that the risk of infertility over a 12 month period was 55 percent higher among women who drank as little as one cup of coffee per day.

Those who drank up to 3 cups per day had an almost 100 percent decrease in their ability to get pregnant. Those who drank more than 3 cups a day saw their infertility odds rise to a whopping 176 percent in just one year!

Perhaps even more disturbing is research out of McGill University in Canada. Here doctors learned that just two to three cups of coffee per day could double the risk of miscarriage.

The good news: If you are hooked on caffeine – and just can't get through the day without it - switching from coffee to tea may not only help quench your need but also increase your fertility.

Indeed, in one study published in the American Journal of Health, doctors noted that women who drank more than 1/2 cup of caffeinated tea daily were twice as likely to get pregnant as those who drank no tea!

While we're still not certain why the caffeine in coffee appears to be more detrimental to fertility than that which is found in tea, my personal theory is that additional compounds within the tea may be what's really behind the fertility boost - and they also be neutralizing some of the negative effects of the caffeine.

Either way, limiting your coffee consumption while trying to get pregnant may give your fertility a small but important boost.

One more important note: For many women coffee is often paired with cigarettes - in fact, for some it's almost automatic to "light up" each time they have a mug of java in their hands!

Much like the combo of alcohol and cigarettes, combining caffeine and cigarettes also amplifies the negative health effects of both.

So, if you can, cut out both. If you can't, try not to have them together.

Instead of coffee, try a steamy mug of hot chocolate. The caffeine load is much lower, plus you'll get a dose of fertility-boosting polyphenols from the cocoa!

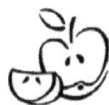

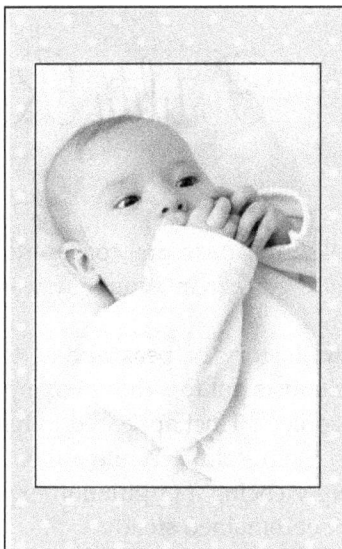

Fertility Robber # 3: Peas!

Although peas are considered a healthy food, when it comes to getting pregnant, you may want to push them off the plate! Why?

The history of peas and fertility goes back as far as 1949, when scientists put together two important observations. The first was that people of Tibet appeared to have one of the most stable populations in the world. While other countries in the same region were experiencing a population explosion, the number of people within Tibet remained steady.

The second was that peas were a staple in their diet. That made researchers question whether or not the two could be related – and that working somewhat like birth control, peas might actually play a role in preventing a population explosion.

As time went on research showed this may in fact be true. Indeed, scientists identified a natural chemical found in peas known as m-xylohydroquinone. In studies conducted in India this compound was made into capsules and and tested as a contraceptive. The result: It was found to decrease sperm production by some 50% and it reduced pregnancy rates by up to 60%.

In the United States studies conducted in the 1990's at the University of Illinois helped further establish the fertility–reducing effects of this compound – which is now under research as a natural form of contraception!

If peas are among your favorite foods – don't fret. A portion or two a week is not likely to harm your fertility –and the benefits as a source of plant protein could actually help. But if you or your partner eats them every day I definitely suggest cutting down to no more than two servings per week.

Fertility Robber # 4 : Diet Soda & Designer Sugars

Whether you drink coffee, tea or soda, you may be wondering whether or not beverages sweetened with the so-called artificial "designer sugars" - products such as Nutra Sweet, Splenda, asulfamine-K, and others - can be harmful to fertility.

And I have to be honest with you and say this is a tough question to answer.

What I can tell you is that the artificial sweetener known as saccharin is something you must avoid. Studies presented to the American College of Nutrition reported that this non-nutritive sweetener may not be safe to consume either while trying to get pregnant or once you are pregnant.

As to the other sugar substitutes, the truth is, we just don't know. Certainly, there are no medical studies linking any of these products directly to fertility or, once you do conceive, to the health of your baby. But that said, it's also important to note that it's against the law to conduct studies on pregnant women, so the truth is we really don't have the kind of solid evidence that I and many other doctors would like in order to get behind the use of sugar substitutes 100 percent.

So while I can't say for sure they will harm your fertility, based on what we know now, I also can't promise that they won't.

So, if you want to continue using your sugar substitutes, remember that moderation is the key.

As such, I would limit consumption to no more than two servings of artificial sweetener a day – and when possible avoid them completely. Also remember, that it's not just the sweeteners you add to beverages or cereals that count, but also those found in prepared beverages, candy, yogurt, ice cream, and other artificially sweetened products. So, be sure to "do the math"!

Most important, don't obsess over your choices and don't worry. Stress and anxiety is likely to play a bigger role in harming your fertility so it's important that you don't fret about the smaller things in life!

Sweet and Natural?

The latest designer sugar to hit the market is SUSTA - a proprietary blend of several natural ingredients including a "sweet" fiber known as "inulin", and fructose or "fruit sugar."

Although SUSTA claims to be "all natural", since they don't list all their individual ingredients, it's difficult to say for sure. Moreover, since there is no government watchdog agency determining use of the word "natural" in any food product, there are no standards the company must meet in order to make the claim.

That said, if SUSTA does turn out to be as natural as their ads say, then certainly it could be an important alternative for those looking to cut sugar from their diet.

Keep in mind, however, that no safety testing of SUSTA has been performed in regard to it's effects on either fertility or pregnancy.

Fertility Robber # 5: Sugar & High Fructose Corn Syrup

There is perhaps nothing more refreshing after a workout class or day in the park than a icy glass of soda or fruit juice. And, in fact, if you are trying to avoid artificial sweeteners then you might be tempted to switch to beverages and foods sweetened with "the real thing", which of course is sugar.

While in some instances this might be a good idea, when it comes to your fertility there are some important concerns. Indeed, a number of studies show that consuming large amounts of sugar – be it in soda, fruit juice, candy or other snack foods – can be harmful to your overall health, and maybe your fertility. This includes increasing your risk of both insulin resistance and type 2 diabetes.

Indeed, while it was once believed that there was no link between dietary sugar consumption and the onset of these conditions, today we know that a diet high in refined, "simple" carbohydrates (which are metabolized as sugar) as well as refined sugar itself, can increase your risk of both these conditions – and in doing so, make it much harder to get pregnant.

Additionally, drinking lots of sugar-laden soft drinks or even fruit juices can also increase your risk of a vaginal yeast infection , a condition which changes the pH or acid level of your vaginal fluids. This, in turn, can be harmful to sperm - sometimes even killing them before they can get through to your reproductive system.

If you find you are plagued with recurring yeast infections, cutting down on sugar might be very helpful.

But there is also something else you need to know about "sweet" foods. While some sodas, juices and snack foods are sweetened with "real " sugar, increasingly manufacturers are replacing sugar with a cheaper sweetener known as high fructose corn syrup. It's made by changing the glucose in cornstarch to a product that is part fructose and part glucose.

But while the method of making corn syrup may sound simple, trust me when I tell you this is not something Grandma would have cooked up on her kitchen stove. In fact, the process is actually quite complex, involving lots of chemicals and other somewhat murky ingredients necessary to change these molecules into a sweetening agent.

It also requires chemical "rearranging" of several key enzymes, all of which impact the way your body processes these ingredients. Indeed, while natural sugar can be metabolized by every cell in the body, high fructose corn syrup is processed much like alcohol or even some medications - taking place in the liver. And therein lies some of the health concerns.

In fact, studies show that animals fed diets rich in high fructose corn syrup were found to have liver damage similar to what occurs from alcohol abuse! While other studies have been less conclusive, still the evidence has me and many doctors putting a red flag on those foods that contain high fructose corn syrup.

From a fertility standpoint the most disturbing evidence of all recently came to light when some studies showed that certain sources of high fructose corn syrup contained significant amounts of mercury, a heavy metal that even in small amounts can have some devastating health effects, particularly on children. My personal concern is that if you are consuming   large amounts of high fructose corn syrup at the time when conception occurs, your unborn baby may be affected.

So, how do you satisfy your sweet tooth without harming your fertility or your baby? As with most things in like, moderation is key. If you want to err on the side of caution, go light and easy on all sugar consumption, but especially foods sweetened with high fructose corn syrup. And doing so may be easier than you think.

You can, for example, use fresh fruit to sweeten your cereal or yogurt, and replace the jelly on your P&J sandwich with a fruit puree.

Since many sodas and even fruit juices can contain up to six tablespoons of sugar and even more corn syrup in a single serving , dilute them with lots of ice or some plain club soda so you consume less. You won't taste much of a difference and you could easily cut your sugar consumption in half.

Essentially, try to cut down how and when you can.

High fructose corn syrup is often lurking in products you might never think to check - like breads, frozen vegetable dishes, even some frozen pizzas! But many manufacturers are also making an effort to cut out high fructose corn syrup, so it pays to take a few extra minutes while shopping to read labels.

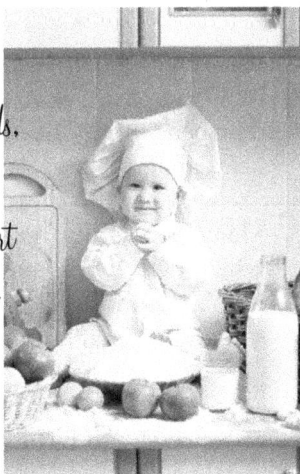

Fertility Robber # 6: Food Preservatives

Among the most common food preservatives is MSG – short for monosodium glutamate. It's also used as a flavor enhancer in many frozen foods (particularly frozen fish entrees), lots of Asian cuisines, and many snack foods, such as flavored potato chips and crackers.

While other additives – including certain flavorings or colorings, as well as other taste enhancers - can also contain glutamate (such as malted barley, caramel flavoring, even some milk powders), MSG contains about 78% – the highest found in any compound.

For those who are sensitive to the glutamate compound, ingesting MSG can lead to a variety of symptoms including hot flashes, diarrhea, hives, headaches, joint pain, dizziness, and temporary heart abnormalities .

Many people also experience something called MSG Syndrome – which results in a temporary (but none-the-less scary) sensation of numbness in the face and head and tightness in the chest that can sometimes even mimic the signs of a heart attack.

Although the evidence linking MSG to any specific health concerns or especially to fertility is not abundant, what we do have is quite startling.

In research conducted by Northeastern University it was suggested that consuming high amounts of MSG before mating reduced the chance of getting pregnant by a whopping 50%! Moreover, when pregnancy did occur, offspring were shorter, with males having smaller testicles.

In other research, animals fed MSG later developed lesions in their hypothalamus gland, an area of the brain which is not only linked to ovulation, but also appetite. In this study the animals exhibited signs of leptin resistance, a hormone that has been shown to influence hunger and satiation - in other words, how full we feel. This theory also proved true in humans when a recent study found that those folks who regularly consumed foods with the highest concentrations of MSG were more likely to become obese.

The common food additive known as MSG has been shown in studies to cause weight gain - which in turn can interfere with your fertility.

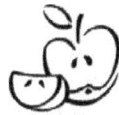

The point here is that if you are already having ovulatory problems, and most especially if you are struggling with a weight problem (which can impact fertility) this might be one food additive you want to avoid.

Unfortunately however that may be easier said than done. While manufacturers are required to list MSG on all food labels, many food purists argue that this ingredient is often "hidden" in products by listing it under an alternate name. Indeed, some alternates by which

MSG is known can include : hydrolyzed vegetable protein, (HVP), autolyzed or hydrolyzed plant protein (HPP or APP), autolyzed yeast, sodium caseinate, Calcium caseinate, and numerous other terms.

So, if you want to avoid MSG completely, check the labels for these other compounds. The foods most commonly known to contain some form of MSG include prepared frozen fish, canned fish, prepared frozen chicken, and canned soups.

More Alphabet Soup: BHA

While you're reading those labels looking for MSG, you might also want to check for another common preservative known as BHA. Found in a variety of baked goods and snack foods , there is some evidence to show that it may mimic the effects of estrogen, which in high enough quantities could cause a hormone imbalance that is significant enough to impair fertility.

Because this entire area of study is still in the early stages, definitive studies linking BHA - or any food additive or preservative - specifically to fertility problems is preliminary at best. In the case of MSG there is no clear published evidence that it impacts fertility in humans. However, it has been my experience that studies which indicate an impact on animal fertility frequently turn out to be turn in humans as well, so for me the research remains a concern.

Indeed it is my personal suggestion that in order to maximize your fertility it is wise to reduce or avoid consumption of foods high in MSG or BHA during the time you are trying to conceive. And certainly you should reduce or avoid them completely once you do become pregnant.

CHAPTER NINE

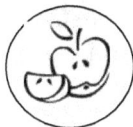

Your Personal
Fertility Food Guide

What To Eat To Get Pregnant Fast!

By now I hope you have come to realize all the many connections between what you eat and your fertility - and just how important you daily diet can be to your reproductive health.

It's not just a matter of getting your daily dose of vitamins and minerals - though that is important. It's also a matter of combining your foods in a way that helps balance your hormones and give your body the optimal level of energy necessary to ensure that every aspect of the reproductive process functions not just normally, but at peak capacity.

This means not just your ovaries and your uterus, but all of the biochemistry involved, including your brain chemistry.

But as I mentioned in the beginning of this book, I never believed in giving my patients a structured, rigid diet to follow – or in telling them they "must" eat certain foods while avoiding others. I've never known that kind of eating plan to be successful - whether you're trying to lose weight or enhance fertility!

The approach that has worked best for thousands of my patients over the years is to simply provide them with the pertinent information on the foods that science shows are beneficial to fertility, and allow them to create their own meal plans, based on the foods like to eat.

And that is what you will find in this final chapter:A Fertility Food Guide meant to help you create the personalized meal plans that are right for you.

Of course for some of you, it's not just the foods you choose, but also the amount of calories they contain that also matters. This is true whether you need to gain or lose weight in order to increase your chance for getting pregnant.

So to help you in this respect I've made sure to include the calorie counts and serving sizes of each food in the following Fertility Food Index, along with a fertility-based caloric intake guide.

That said, it's also important to note that I've also never been a doctor who believed in rigid daily calorie counting as a way to achieve weight goals. And that's because I've never known a patient who gained or lost weight based on what she ate in a single day!

Instead I have always suggested to my patients to look at their *food intake averages*, usually over a 7 day period. This works for two important reasons.

First, if you happen to eat more on a particular day (maybe you are extra hungry, expecting your period or have an event to attend), you won't panic just because you went over your caloric intake for that day.

And that is because you know you can always use the following day or two to balance out your weekly caloric plan.

So, for example, if you are on a 2,000 calorie a day diet, but on day two of the week you eat 2400 calories - don't panic! On days three and four you simply cut back to 1800 calories a day. If you do, then by day five you're right back on track!

A little later in this book you'll find my suggested weekly caloric intake guides for gaining, losing, or maintaining your best fertility weight. Using these numbers as a guide, you can turn to the the calorie counts in the Fertility Food Guide to create menus and meal plans that you'll really enjoy.

While calories might be one important consideration when planning your fertility diet, there are others. Among the most important is a food's nutrient "volume". And by that I mean how many fertility nutrients are packed into each bite!

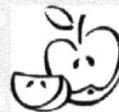

While calories can be one important food factor to consider when planning your diet, it's not the only factor. Among the most important things to consider is a food's nutrient value.

As you read throughout this book, many foods have a particular impact on fertility. Most often that impact is based on the protein and vitamin-mineral content, the antioxidant potential or the amount of phytonutrients it contains. For this reason it's also important that you consider some of your personal, individual fertility needs when choosing what foods to include in your diet.

For example, as you read in an earlier chapter, if you are having problems with ovulation (often indicated by irregular menstrual cycles) then you will need to focus on foods that encourage ovulation, such as low fat red meat, or foods high in complex carbohydrates like whole wheat bread and cereals. And you'll need to make a point of avoiding simple carbohydrates - like white bread and pasta - and not eat too many sweets.

Similarly, if you have been diagnosed with fertility robbing conditions such as endometriosis or PCOs – you'll need to pay attention to the "inflammation ratings" of the foods you choose, focusing on those items that have potent anti-inflammatory effects. (And you'll learn a bit more about how to do that in just a few moments).

What I am really saying here is that you know best what your specific fertility concerns are, so use the information in the Food Index to help guide to the types of foods that will work best for you.

What's more, you may be surprised - or even shocked - to discover how oftentimes making simple substitutions in your daily diet, sometimes even just subbing one brand of your favorite food for another, can make a huge difference in not only your caloric intake, but your intake of fertility boosting nutrients.

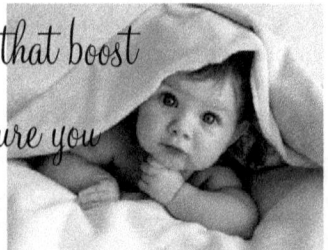

Remember ... the same foods that boost your fertility can also help insure you give birth to a healthier baby!

YOUR PERSONAL FERTILITY FOOD GUIDE

Choose Your Fertility Foods Wisely: What To Look For

When is a piece of fish more than just a piece of fish? Sounds like the start of puzzling riddle, I know!

But the truth is that when it comes to enhancing your fertility, both the benefits and risks associated with certain foods can change dramatically depending on where they originate from and how they are prepared.

Here are some examples to watch out for!

White canned tuna is loaded with fertility-enhancing Omega-3 fatty acids, but *light tuna* has less than half the amount!

Wild salmon is packed with numerous nutrients known to boost fertility, but by comparison *farmed salmon* contains hardly any!

A burger made from *95% lean ground beef* contains just 7 grams of fat; make that burger from *85% lean ground beef,* and you more than double the fat content to a whopping 15 grams!

Roast a chicken breast and you have just 142 calories; *fry that same chicken breast* and you're eating 364 calories!

Fry your foods in canola oil and get a whopper dose of fertility-enhancing omega-3 fatty acids; *fry those same foods in olive oil* and you hardly get any omega 3 at all!

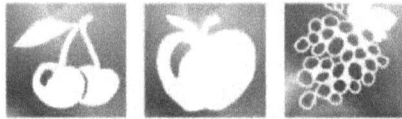

Smart Food - Healthy Food: The Anti-Inflammatory Diet

As you read in an earlier chapter, one factor that can impact not only fertility, but many aspects of your health is inflammation – a kind of body-wide reaction that can occur in response to any number of factors. These include excess body fat (and particularly belly fat) as well as chronic stress, including psychological as well as physiologic stress, some of which develops as a result of poor diet.

In addition to impacting your fertility, inflammation is now thought to be an underlying cause of heart disease, high blood pressure, diabetes and even some cancers - so it's clearly a factor worthy of our attention.

In fact, the impact of inflammation on both general health and specifically on fertility can be so great, it's even measurable in the blood, most often by a test for a protein known as CPR – or C Reactive Protein, a natural compound that rises anytime your body is dealing with inflammation.

For those of you already diagnosed with an inflammation -related condition such as endometriosis or PCOS , then the inflammatory response can not only decrease your fertility, but also worsen some of your symptoms. But even if you don't have these conditions, the latest research shows that to some extent the health of all women is affected by inflammation– with "unexplained infertility" frequently the diagnosis for those already affected.

So what does all this have to do with diet – and specifically a "Fertility Diet"?

One of the more outstanding nutritional discoveries of recent years has been the recognition of the way in which certain foods can both encourage and discourage the production of inflammatory chemicals in the body. In essence we have learned which foods have the ability to create or exacerbate inflammation , and which ones calm down or neutralize inflammation, and maybe even undo some of the damage that has already occurred And no where is this more true than when it comes to your fertility.

Indeed,   studies have shown – and my own personal patient-centered research has proven to me personally - that certain anti-inflammatory foods have the ability to promote fertility and encourage a quicker pregnancy while inflammatory foods can slow down the entire process. In some women they may even play a role in preventing pregnancy from occurring at all!

So how do you know which foods fall into which category?

Well for a long time it was really a matter of "hit and miss". Through experimentation and some personal experience we slowly began to weed out which foods appeared to be inflammatory and which ones were likely to calm body responses. While the system seemed to be working, it was cumbersome, and difficult to personalize for each woman.

Then, a few years ago something quite wonderful occurred. Thanks to a researcher and nutritionist named Monica Reinagel, the entire process of identifying the inflammatory potential of foods became simplified - to the point where the concept could be put to use by almost anyone!

Indeed, after spending years researching this area of nutrition, Ms. Reinagel was able to narrow the inflammatory process down to just 20 specific nutrients -- factors she discovered make a difference in every single food where they are present.

Using this information, and data on the nutrient value of hundreds of foods, Ms. Reinagel developed a brand new and very unique food rating system – a way of not only measuring, but also identifying the inflammatory potential of some 1500 of the most common foods.

She named her system **The IF Rating-** short for **Inflammatory Response Rating and** she published her findings in a groundbreaking book titled "The Inflammation Factor".

If you are interested in learning more about inflammatory foods, and particularly if you have been diagnosed with any inflammatory condition including PCOS, endometriosis, Lupus or rheumatoid arthritis, I strongly advise you to pick up a copy of this eye-opening book.

In the meantime, however, based on Ms. Reinagel's research and findings, I have been able to feature the IF ratings for each of the foods I recommend in the Fertility Food Index featured in the next chapter. So, as a part of each food's nutrient profile you will also find the Inflammation Rating for that food - including an explanation of what that rating represents.

According to Ms. Reinagel's system, foods with a "negative" IF rating (indicated on the profile by a "minus" sign) are considered to be *inflammatory* . And the higher the number, the more inflammatory the food is.

Foods with a positive IF rating (indicated by the lack of a "minus sign") means they are *anti-inflammatory* - and again, the higher the number, the more anti-inflammatory properties that food has.

What's also important to note is that the ratings are also considered to be dose-responsive. And by that I mean the more of these foods you eat, the higher the ratings go. So, for example, while a teaspoon of corn oil may be "mildly inflammatory" a cup of this same oil turns it into a food that is "highly inflammatory".

Of course the good news is that the opposite also applies. If three ounces of wild salmon is "moderately anti-inflammatory", then nine ounces can easily be "strongly anti-inflammatory".

This is important to know for two reasons. First, it means that the more "good" foods you eat the more protection you get. But it also means that even "cutting down" on the not-so-good foods can have an important positive impact on your health and your fertility.

Balancing Your Fertility Food Equation

What's important to note, however, is that you do not have to create a diet based solely on "anti-inflammatory" foods. In fact, doing so would not even be healthy. Why?

Simply put, the inflammatory rating of a food is only one measure of its worth - and quite honestly there may be some foods which, while they are considered somewhat inflammatory, might still possess nutrients and compounds that are important to your health and your fertility in other ways.

In fact, red meat is a great example. While it's considered to be somewhat "inflammatory", in moderate amounts it can actually give your fertility a boost, particularly if you are having problems with ovulation. So, excluding it from your diet would not be a good idea.

The same is true for many foods, including many types of fruits and vegetables.

The point is to use these IF ratings to create a better "balanced" meal plan, with enough anti-inflammatory foods to offset those with a high inflammation rating that may be important to eat for other reasons.

Indeed, it is this balance between the two food types that is going to give your health, but particularly our fertility, the greatest boost.

Moreover, accomplishing this is simple if you stop to consider the IF ratings of the foods you choose and look to balance the pluses and the minuses.

For example, on the days you choose to eat a food with a higher inflammatory rating, be certain to also include at least one meal that is based in anti-inflammatory foods.

Keeping this balance in mind will allow you to eat more of the foods you love, with less fear and worry, and still impact your fertility in a positive way.

Remember ...

if a food has a "negative" IF rating that means it is inflammatory - which may have some negative effects on fertility in some women.

If a food has a "positive" IF rating, then it is considered anti-inflammatory and may have a helpful even healing influence on fertility.

As a guideline, nutrition experts suggest you aim for 50 or more positive IF anti-inflammatory rating points in your diet every day. You should also try to minimize IF inflammatory points .

The Sweet Truth About Getting Pregnant

How Blood Sugar Affects Your Fertility

When it comes to creating your personalized fertility food program, there is one more number within the nutrient value ratings I'm going to ask you to pay attention to. And that is, Glycemic Load Index, which is listed for each food in my Fertility Food Index.

What is this - and why is it important ? Simply put, it's a practical, easy way to determine the impact any food has on your blood sugar.

In short, the Glycemic Load tells you if a certain food will cause your blood sugar, and consequently insulin levels, to rise quickly (indicated by a high number) or if it will little or no impact on either one (as indicated by a low or a negative number).

And how will this information impact your fertility?

As you read earlier in this book a diet high in foods that cause an quick and immediate rise in blood sugar can, over time, cause your cells to become "resistant" to the effects of insulin. When this occurs, sugars can't be removed from your blood stream as quickly or effectively as they need to be.

Moreover, when this goes on for a long enough period of time, the hormonal network necessary for conception can become disrupted, and your fertility can suffer.

One way to avoid all these problems is to eat more foods with a "low" glycemic load - foods rated at 10 or less . Also important is to eat fewer foods with a "high " glycemic load, rated at 20 or more.

To help you make the right choices, I've included the Glycemic Load Index for every food listed in the Fertility Food Index. Whenever possible the actual glycemic load data is presented; in foods where this information is not available a mathematical formula was used to calculate the nutrient value of the food and approximate the Glycemic Load Index.

In using this information, however, keep in mind that most nutritionists now agree that aiming for 100 or less "glycemic load points" per day is a healthy way to eat and important way to promote and protect your fertility!

Having your cake ...
and eating it too!

By making simple ingredient substitutions - such as switching out white flour for whole wheat and cutting the sugar in your recipe by just 1/3 - you can lower the glycemic load on treats like brownies!

A Final Word:
Eat Healthy, Be Happy, Don't Worry!

In the last section of this book - which starts on the following page-you will discover the final pieces of information necessary to customize a personal fertility food plan: The nutrient and other fertility values of more than 200 of the best foods known to boost fertility.

If you use it wisely, you can not only boost your fertility and get pregnant faster, but also take steps to improve your overall health - something which will bring you many benefits for decades to come.

I hope that this special food guide, together will all the information present in this book, will provide you with not only help and information, but also inspiration to go forward with your dreams of motherhood - and to never give up!

But my personal "take home" message - from me to you - is simply this: Eat as healthfully as you can and then don't worry! While your diet can certainly play an important role in helping you get pregnant, if you are filled with worry and fear over what you are eating, the resulting stress will only negate the wonderful benefits of a healthy diet!

Certainly, it's important to heed lifestyle and dietary precautions when and how you can. But what's equally important is that you remain positive about your ability to get pregnant. In fact, in addition to eating healthy the two most important things you can do to prepare your body for pregnancy is to remain optimistic, and reduce stress in your life.

So, above all - *be happy and don't worry!* The magic of pregnancy will happen for you!

CHAPTER TEN:

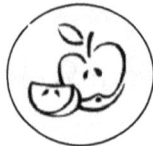

Your Fertility Food Guide Index

How To Choose The Fertility Foods That Are Right For You!

Choosing The Foods That Will Help You Get Pregnant Fast:

How To Use This Guide

The Foods you will find in the following guide represent not only what the latest research indicates can be beneficial for fertility, but also those foods that I have recommended throughout my 30 years of helping thousands of women get pregnant and deliver happy,smart, and healthy babies!

Certainly there are other "fertility foods" - many of them endemic to cultures and ethnic groups around the globe and steeped in both folklore and local legend. And in many instances, there is much anecdotal evidence that they do indeed work. To this end please know that the following lists of foods is by no means the definitive guide to fertility boosting foods.

That said, the foods that *are* featured in this guide are what I believe -and what my patients have proven - to be key players when it comes to encouraging a quick and healthy pregnancy.

 However, when choosing the items that will make up your Personal Fertility Food Plan, it's also important to include as much variety in your diet as you can. While some foods are high in certain key nutrients, they may be low in others, so it usually takes a "team approach" to achieve strong nutritional balance.

To this end, I not only agree with the recommendations of the new FDA Food Pyramid, but I have used these values to create my very own Fertility Food Pyramid - a visualization of everything you have learned in this book thus far . And you will find it on the next page.

My suggestion is to use it as a base for selecting the foods in your personal fertility plan.

Ice
Cream

Healthy
Beverages –
Like Green Tea
Plus Dark Chocolate

Healthy
Oils

Healthy
Fats

Vegetable
Protein

Nuts

Low Fat
Dairy

Whole Grains

Fish, Poultry, &
Lean Beef

Organic Fruits –
especially berries

Fresh Vegetables
especially cruciferous type

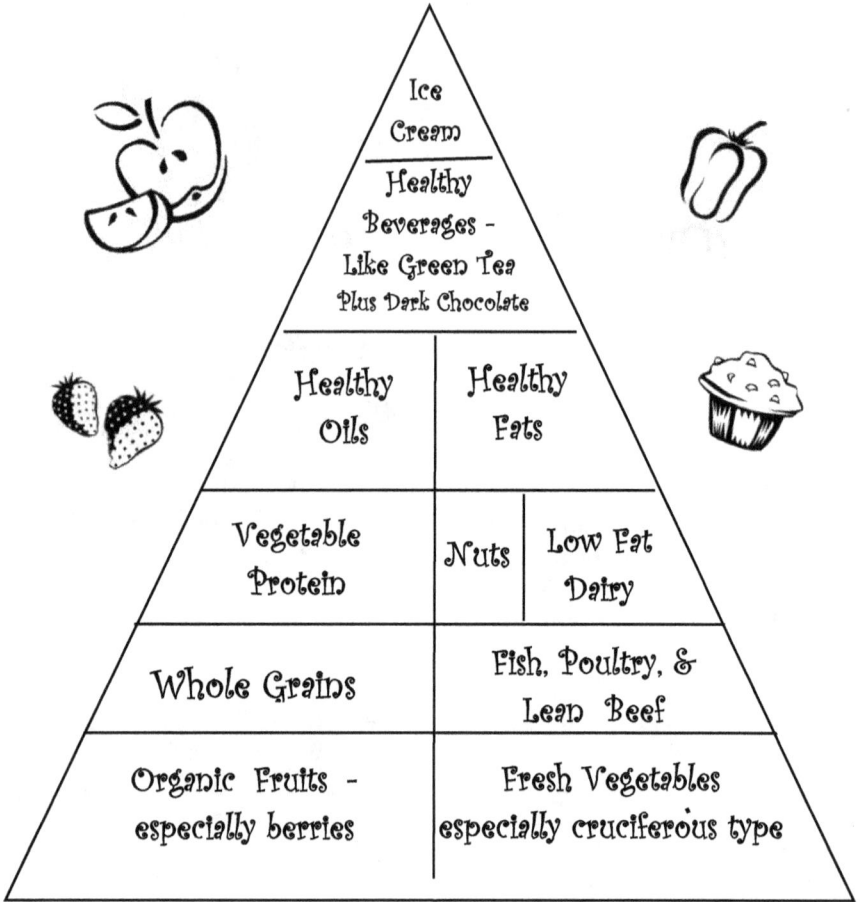

Your Fertility Food Pyramid

The food groups that can help encourage fertility and help you
get pregnant faster and easier!

Part of this new pyramid is the suggestion to include at least 3 to 4 fruits and vegetables in your daily diet - and more if you can. It's also important to avoid as much saturated fat as possible, and to keep sugars and processed foods to a minimum.

In fact, to this end I have purposefully omitted a "dessert"category, with hopes that you will instead satisfy your "sweet tooth" with the many luscious fruits on the list. When this isn't quite enough, I urge you to check our website at **GettingPregantNow.org,** where you'll soon find recipes for delicious and healthful "fertility desserts" - including our famous "Fertility Brownies"!

Additionally, I know that for some of you, weight is also a concern, and that you may need to either gain or lose a few pounds in order to maximize your chances of getting pregnant. So to help put you on the right path - and to help those of you at the right weight to maintain it - at the end of the food section you will also find some helpful fertility weight management tips and tools.

These include:
- A Fertility Height & Weight Chart
- BMI - Body Mass Index Chart
- Fertility BMI Risk Factor Chart
- 7 Day Caloric Intake Guide

Together with the Fertility Food Guide Index these tools can help you not only plan the meals that will help you get pregnant faster and easier, but also the meals that will improve your health on all fronts!

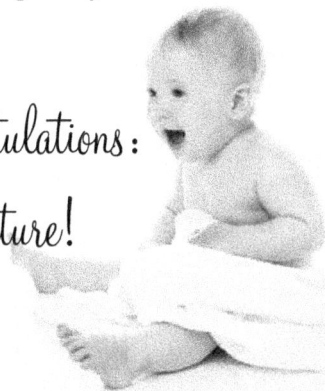

So bon appetite and congratulations:

A baby is in your near future!

Fertility Food List Index

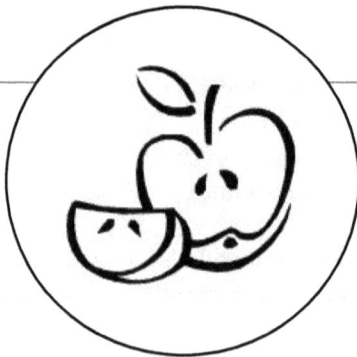

The Fertility Fruits

Apples
Serving: 1 apple (3") with skin.
Calories: 95
Protein: 0
Fiber: 4 grams
Carbohydrates: 25 grams
Fat: 0
Sugars: 19 grams
Glycemic Load Index: 5
Inflammatory Rating: -30 (mildly inflammatory)
Key Vitamins & Minerals: C (14% of RDA)

Apricots
Serving: 3 apricots (totaling 4 oz.)
Calories: 51
Protein: 0
Fiber: 3 grams
Carbohydrates: 11.8 grams
Fat: 0
Sugars: 9 grams
Glycemic Load Index: 3
Inflammatory Rating: 1   mildly anti-inflammatory
Key Vitamins & Minerals: A (13% of RDA per apricot

Avacados (California)
Serving: 1 without skin (6 oz)
Calories: 227
Protein: 3 grams
Fiber: 9.3 grams
Carbohydrates: 12 grams
Fat: 21 grams (3 grams saturated)
Sugars: 0 mg
Glycemic Load Index: 3
Inflammatory Rating: 107 (moderately anti-

Bananas
Serving: 1 medium
Calories: 105
Protein: 1 gram
Fiber: 3 grams
Carbohydrates: 27 grams
Fat: 0
Sugars: 14 grams
Glycemic Load Index: 10
Inflammatory Rating: - 60 (mildly inflammatory)
Key Vitamins & Minerals: B6(22% of RDA), C (17% of RDA) Potassium (12% of RDA).

Blueberries (Wild, from Alaska)
Serving: ½ cup
Calories: 61
Protein: 1 gram
Fiber: 3.5 grams
Carbohydrates: 12 grams
Fat: 1 gram
Sugars: 6 grams
Glycemic Load Index: 4
Inflammatory Rating: N/A
Key Vitamins & Minerals: C (30% of RDA)

Blueberries (regular)
Serving: 1 cup
Calories: 84
Protein: 1 gram
Fiber: 4 grams
Carbohydrates: 21 grams
Fat: 0
Sugars: 15 grams
Glycemic Load Index: 6
Inflammatory Rating: - 28 (mildly inflammatory)
Key Vitamins & Minerals: C (24% of RDA); K (36% of RDA)

Cantaloupe
Serving: ½ melon (9.5 oz)
Calories: 95
Protein: 2.5 grams
Fiber: 2.5 grams
Carbohydrates: 22.4 grams
Fat: .8 grams
Sugars: 21 grams
Glycemic Load Index: 7
Inflammatory Rating: 238 (moderately anti-inflammatory)
Key Vitamins & Minerals: A (180% of RDA); C (160% of RDA); Folate (15% of RDA) B6 (10% of RDA)

Cherries (Sweet, with pits)
Serving: 1 cup
Calories: 87
Protein: 1 gram
Fiber: 3 grams
Carbohydrates: 22 grams
Fat: 0
Sugars: 18 grams
Glycemic Load Index: 7
Inflammatory Rating: - 47 (mildly inflammatory)
Key Vitamins & Minerals: C (16% of RDA);

Cranberries (unsweetened)
Serving: 1 cup
Calories: 46
Protein: 0
Fiber: 5 grams
Carbohydrates: 12 grams
Fat: 0
Sugars: 4 grams
Glycemic Load Index: 2
Inflammatory Rating: -4 (mildly inflammatory)
Key Vitamins & Minerals: C (22% of RDA);

Grapes (Red or Green)
Serving: 1 cup
Calories: 104
Protein: 1 gram
Fiber: 1 gram
Carbohydrates: 27 grams
Fat: 0
Sugars: 23 grams
Glycemic Load Index: 9
Inflammatory Rating: - 56 (mildly inflammatory)
Key Vitamins & Minerals : C (27% of RDA)

Grapefruit
Serving: ½
Calories: 52
Protein: 1 gram
Fiber: 2 grams
Carbohydrates: 13 grams
Fat: 0
Sugars: 8 grams
Glycemic Load Index: 4
Inflammatory Rating: 10 (mildly anti-inflammatory)
Key Vitamins & Minerals: C (64% of RDA); A (28 % of RDA)

Guava
Serving: 1
Calories: 37
Protein: 1 gram
Fiber: 3 grams
Carbohydrates: 8 grams
Fat: 1 grams
Sugars: 5 grams
Glycemic Load Index: 2
Inflammatory Rating: 44 (mildly anti-inflammatory
Key Vitamins & Minerals : C (209% of RDA);

Honey Dew Melon
Serving: 10 melon balls
Calories: 50
Protein: 1 gram
Fiber: 1 gram
Carbohydrates : 13 grams
Fat: 0
Sugars: 11 grams
Glycemic Load Index: 3
Inflammatory Rating: -5 (mildly inflammatory)
Key Vitamins & Minerals: C (41% of RDA).

Nectarine
Serving: 1 medium (2.5")
Calories: 63
Protein: 2 grams
Fiber: 2 grams
Carbohydrates: 15 grams
Fat: 0
Sugars: 11 grams
Glycemic Load Index: 5
Inflammatory Rating: - 26 (mildly inflammatory)
Key Vitamins & Minerals: C (13% of RDA) A (9% of RDA) Niacin (8% of RDA).

Orange
Serving: 1 (2.5 ")
Calories : 65
Protein: 1 gram
Fiber: 3 grams
Carbohydrates: 16 grams
Fat: 0.2 grams
Sugars: 13 grams
Glycemic Load Index: 4
Inflammatory Rating: 4 (mildly anti-inflammatory)
Key Vitamins & Minerals: C (106% of RDA).

Papaya
Serving: 1 medium (5" x 3 ")
Calories: 119
Protein: 2
Fiber: 5
Carbohydrates: 30
Fat: 0
Sugars: 18
Glycemic Load Index: 7
Inflammatory Rating: 71 (mildly anti-inflammatory)
Key Vitamins & Minerals: C (391% of RDA); A (83% of RDA)
Folate (36% of RDA); Potassium (28% of RDA).

Peach
Serving: 1 large (2 3/4")
Calories: 68
Protein: 2 grams
Fiber: 3 grams
Carbohydrates: 17 grams
Fat: 0
Sugars: 15 grams
Glycemic Load Index: 5
Inflammatory Rating: 25 (mildly anti-inflammatory)
Key Vitamins & Minerals: C (19% of RDA) A (11% of RDA)

Pear
Serving: 1 medium
Calories: 103
Protein: 0
Fiber: 6 grams
Carbohydrates: 28 grams
Fat: 0
Sugars: 17 grams
Glycemic Load Index: 6
Inflammatory Rating: -36 (mildly inflammatory)
Key Vitamins & Minerals: C (12% of RDA) K (10% of RDA)
Potassium (6% of RDA).

Raspberries
Serving: 1 cup
Calories: 64
Protein: 1 gram
Fiber: 8 grams
Carbohydrates: 15 grams
Fat: 1 gram
Sugars: 5 grams
Glycemic Load Index: 3
Inflammatory Rating: 1 (mildly anti-inflammatory)
Key Vitamins & Minerals: C (54% of RDA); K (12% of RDA)

Strawberries
Serving: 1 cup of halves
Calories: 49
Protein: 1 gram
Fiber: 3 grams
Carbohydrates: 12 grams
Fat: 0
Sugars: 7 grams
Glycemic Load Index: 3
Inflammatory Rating: 28 (mildly anti-inflammatory)
Key Vitamins & Minerals: C (149% of RDA) Folate (9% of RDA)

Watermelon
Serving: 10 melon balls (1/3 wedge)
Calories: 37
Protein: 1 gram
Fiber: 0
Carbohydrates: 9 grams
Fat: 0
Sugars: 8 grams
Glycemic Load Index: 3
Inflammatory Rating: - 6 (mildly inflammatory)

The Fertility Veggies

Artichokes (Jerusalem)
Serving: 1 cup slices
Calories: 109
Protein: 3 grams
Fiber: 0
Carbohydrates: 26 grams
Fat: 0
Sugars: 14 grams
Glycemic Load Index: 11
Inflammatory Rating: -74 (mildly inflammatory)
Key Vitamins & Minerals: C (10% of RDA) Iron (28% of RDA)

Asparagus
Serving: 1 cup
Calories: 27
Protein: 3 grams
Fiber: 3 grams
Carbohydrates:
Fat: 0
Sugars: 3 grams
Glycemic Load Index: 3
Inflammatory Rating: 26 (mildly anti-inflammatory)
Key Vitamins & Minerals:

Beans
Serving Size: 1 cup
Calories : 34
Protein (2 grams)
Fiber (4 grams)
Carbohydrates: 8 grams
Fat: 0
Sugars (2 grams)
Glycemic Load Index (3
Inflammatory Rating: 8 (mildly anti-inflammatory
Key Vitamins & Minerals: C (30% of RDA) A (15% of

Beans (Baked)
Serving: 1 cup
Calories: 239
Protein: 12 grams
Fiber: 10 grams
Carbohydrates: 54 grams
Fat: 1 gram
Sugars: 20 grams
Glycemic Load Index: 19
Inflammatory Rating: - 103 (mildly inflammatory)
Key Vitamins & Minerals: A (5% of RDA); Iron (17% of RDA)

Beans (Kidney, boiled, no salt)
Serving: 1 cup
Calories: 225
Protein: 15 grams
Fiber: 11 grams
Carbohydrates: 40 grams
Fat: 1 gram
Sugars: 1 gram
Glycemic Load Index: 15
Inflammatory Rating: -55 (mildly inflammatory)
Key Vitamins & Minerals: C (4% of RDA); Iron (22% of RDA)

Beans (Lima)
Serving: 1 cup (boiled, no salt)
Calories: 216
Protein: 15 grams
Fiber: 13 grams
Carbohydrates: 39 grams
Fat: 1 gram
Sugars: 5 grams
Glycemic Load Index: 14
Inflammatory Rating: -61 (mildly inflammatory)
Key Vitamins & Minerals: Iron (25% of RDA)

Broccoli
Serving: 1 cup chopped (raw)
Calories: 31
Protein: 3 grams
Fiber: 2 grams
Carbohydrates: 6 grams
Fat: 0
Sugars: 2 grams
Glycemic Load Index: 3
Inflammatory Rating: 53 (mildly anti-inflammatory)
Key Vitamins & Minerals: C (135% of RDA) A (11% of RDA)

Butternut Squash
Serving: 1 cup (cooked without salt)
Calories: 82
Protein: 2 grams
Fiber: 0
Carbohydrates: 22 grams
Fat: 0
Sugars: 2 grams
Glycemic Load Index: 8
Inflammatory Rating: 165 (moderately anti-inflammatory)
Key Vitamins & Minerals: A (457% of RDA) C (52% of RDA)

Cabbage (Green or Red)
Serving: 1 cup (Raw)
Calories: 28 (approximately)
Protein: 1 gram
Fiber: 2 grams
Carbohydrates: 5 to 7 grams
Fat: 0
Sugars: 3 grams
Glycemic Load Index: 2
Inflammatory Rating: 27 (mildly anti-inflammatory)

Cabbage (Chinese)
Serving: 1 cup raw (shredded)
Calories: 9
Protein: 1 gram
Fiber: 1 gram
Carbohydrates: 2 grams
Fat: 0
Sugars:1 gram
Glycemic Load Index: 1
Inflammatory Rating: 63 (mildly anti-inflammatory)
Key Vitamins & Minerals: A (63% of RDA); C (52% of RDA)

Carrots
Serving: 1 medium (raw)
Calories: 25
Protein: 1 gram
Fiber: 2 grams
Carbohydrates: 6 grams
Fat: 0
Sugars: 3 grams
Glycemic Load Index: 2
Inflammatory Rating: 99 (mildly anti-inflammatory)
Key Vitamins & Minerals: A (204% of RDA)

Cauliflower
Serving: 1 cup (raw)
Calories: 25
Protein: 2 grams
Fiber: 3 grams
Carbohydrates: 5 grams
Fat: 0
Sugars: 2 grams
Glycemic Load Index: 2
Inflammatory Rating: 18 (mildly anti-inflammatory)
Key Vitamins & Minerals: C (77% of RDA)

Celery
Serving: 1 medium stalk (7-8")
Calories: 6
Protein: 0
Fiber:1 gram
Carbohydrates: 1 gram
Fat: 0
Sugars: 1 gram
Glycemic Load Index: 0
Inflammatory Rating: 5 (mildly anti-inflammatory)
Key Vitamins & Minerals: A (4% of RDA)

Chickpeas (Garbanzo Beans)
Serving: 1 cup (boiled, no salt)
Calories: 269
Protein: 15 grams
Fiber: 12 grams
Carbohydrates: 45 grams
Fat: 4 grams
Sugars: 8 grams
Glycemic Load Index: 17
Inflammatory Rating: –70 (mildly inflammatory)
Key Vitamins & Minerals: C (4% of RDA) ; Iron (26% of RDA).

Garlic
Serving: 1 clove, 1 cup chopped (raw)
Calories: 6 ; 203
Protein: 9 grams
Fiber: 0 grams; 3 grams
Carbohydrates: 1 gram ; 45 grams
Fat: 0 gram ; 1 gram
Sugars: 0 grams ; 1 gram
Glycemic Load Index: 0; 22
Inflammatory Rating: 107 ; 4,863 (strongly anti-inflammatory)
Key Vitamins & Minerals: C (71% of RDA - for one cup)

Kale
Serving: 1 cup chopped
Calories: 33
Protein: 2 grams
Fiber: 1 gram
Carbohydrates: 7 grams
Fat: 0
Sugars: 0
Glycemic Load Index: 3
Inflammatory Rating: 257 (strongly anti-inflammatory)
Key Vitamins & Minerals: A (206% of RDA) C (134% of RDA)

Lentils
Serving: 1 cup (boiled, no salt)
Calories: 230
Protein: 18 grams
Fiber: 16 grams
Carbohydrates:
Fat: 1 gram
Sugars: 4 grams
Glycemic Load Index: 13
Inflammatory Rating: - 15 (mildly inflammatory)
Key Vitamins & Minerals: C (5% of RDA); Iron (37% of RDA)

Lettuce
Serving: 1 cup shredded
Calories: 5
Protein: 0
Fiber: 0
Carbohydrates: 1 gram
Fat: 0
Sugars: 0
Glycemic Load Index: 1
Inflammatory Rating: 48 (mildly anti-inflammatory)
Key Vitamins & Minerals: A (53% of RDA) C (11% of RDA)

Onions
Serving: 1 cup chopped
Calories: 64
Protein: 2 grams
Fiber: 3 grams
Carbohydrates: 15 grams
Fat: 0
Sugars: 7 grams
Glycemic Load Index: 5
Inflammatory Rating: 374 (strongly anti-
inflammatory) Key Vitamins & Minerals: C (20% of
RDA)

Potatoes -Baked
Serving: 1 large (3-4")
Calories: 278
Protein: 7 grams
Fiber: 7 grams
Carbohydrates: 63 grams
Fat: 0
Sugars: 4 grams
Glycemic Load Index: 29
Inflammatory Rating: 179 (moderately inflammatory)
Key Vitamins & Minerals: C (48% of RDA)

Potatoes (Boiled)
Serving: 1 medium (2.5")
Calories: 118
Protein: 3 grams
Fiber: 2 grams
Carbohydrates: 27 grams
Fat: 0
Sugars: 1 gram
Glycemic Load Index: 12
Inflammatory Rating: - 78 mildly inflammatory

Pumpkin
Serving: 1 cup (cubbed)
Calories: 30
Protein: 1 gram
Fiber: 1 gram
Carbohydrates: 8 grams
Fat: 0
Sugars: 2 grams
Glycemic Load Index: 3
Inflammatory Rating: 65 (mildly anti-inflammatory)
Key Vitamins & Minerals: A (171% of RDA); C (51% of RDA)

Red Peppers
Serving: 1 cup raw (chopped)
Calories: 46
Protein: 1 gram
Fiber: 3 grams
Carbohydrates: 9 grams
Fat: 0
Sugars: 6 grams
Glycemic Load Index: 3
Inflammatory Rating: 126 (mildly anti-inflammatory)
Key Vitamins & Minerals: C (317% of RDA); A (93% of RDA)

Soybeans (Edamame)
Serving: 1 cup
Calories: 130
Protein: 12 grams
Fiber: 6 grams
Carbohydrates: 12 grams
Fat: 6 grams
Sugars: 3 grams
Glycemic Load Index: 4
Inflammatory Rating: N/A
Key Vitamins & Minerals: C (19% of RDA)

Soybeans (green)
Serving: 1 cup (Boiled, no salt)
Calories:
Protein: 22 grams
Fiber: 8 grams
Carbohydrates: 20 grams
Fat: 12 grams
Sugars: n/a
Glycemic Load Index:8
Inflammatory Rating: - 27 (mildly inflammatory)
Key Vitamins & Minerals: C (51% of RDA)

Spinach
Serving: 1 cup
Calories: 7
Protein: 1 gram
Fiber: 1 gram
Carbohydrates: 1 gram
Fat: 0
Sugars: 0
Glycemic Load Index: 0
Inflammatory Rating: 78 (mildly anti-inflammatory)
Key Vitamins & Minerals: A (56% of RDA)

Sweet Potatoes
Serving: 1 (5" long)
Calories: 112
Protein: 2 grams
Fiber: 4 grams
Carbohydrates: 26 grams
Fat: 0
Sugars: 5 grams
Glycemic Load Index: 11
Inflammatory Rating: 160 (moderately anti-
inflammatory) Key Vitamins & Minerals: A (369% of

Tomatoes
Serving: 1 medium (2.5 ")
Calories: 22
Protein: 1 gram
Fiber: 1 gram
Carbohydrates: 5 grams
Fat: 0
Sugars: 3 grams
Glycemic Load Index: 2
Inflammatory Rating: 11 (mildly anti-inflammatory)
Key Vitamins & Minerals:

Winter Squash
Serving: 1 cup cubed (raw)
Calories: 39
Protein: 1 gram
Fiber: 2 grams
Carbohydrates: 10 grams
Fat: 0
Sugars: 3 grams
Glycemic Load Index: 3
Inflammatory Rating: 11 (mildly anti-inflammatory)
Key Vitamins & Minerals: A (32% of RDA) C (24% of RDA)

Yams
Serving: 1 cup (cubed)
Calories:
Protein: 2 grams
Fiber: 6 grams
Carbohydrates: 42 grams
Fat: 0
Sugars: 1 gram
Glycemic Load Index: 18
Inflammatory Rating: -109 (moderately inflammatory)
Key Vitamins & Minerals: C (27% of RDA) B6 (16 % of
RDA); Potassium (26% of RDA); Omega 3 - 12. 2 mg ;
Omega - 6: 68 mg.

Fertility Grains

Barley
Serving:1 ounce (hulled)
Calories: 99
Protein: 3 grams
Fiber: 5 grams
Carbohydrates: 21 grams
Fat: 0
Sugars: 0
Glycemic Load Index:10
Inflammatory Rating: - 64 (mildly inflammatory)
Key Vitamins & Minerals: Thiamin (12% of RDA); Iron (4%RDA)

Buckwheat
Serving: 1 ounce
Calories: 96
Protein: 4 grams
Fiber: 3 grams
Carbohydrates: 20 grams
Fat: 1 gram
Sugars: 0
Glycemic Load Index: 10
Inflammatory Rating: -74 (mildly inflammatory)
Key Vitamins & Minerals: Niacin (10% of RDA)

Oats (Regular, quick, instant, dry)
Serving: 1/3 cup dry
Calories: 102
Protein: 4 grams
Fiber: 3 grams
Carbohydrates: 19 grams
Fat: 2 grams
Sugars: 0
Glycemic Load Index: 11
Inflammatory Rating: -71 (mildly inflammatory)
Key Vitamins & Minerals: Thiamin (8% of RDA)

Quinoa
Serving: 1 ounce (uncooked)
Calories: 103
Protein: 4 grams
Fiber: 2 grams
Carbohydrates: 18 grams
Fat: 2 grams
Sugars: 0
Glycemic Load Index: 10
Inflammatory Rating:- 62 (mildly inflammatory)
Key Vitamins & Minerals: Folate (13% of RDA);Manganese (28% RDA)

Rice (brown)
Serving: 1 cup cooked
Calories: 216
Protein: 5 grams
Fiber: 4 grams
Carbohydrates: 45 grams
Fat: 2 grams
Sugars: 1 gram
Glycemic Load Index: 22
Inflammatory Rating: - 143 (mildly inflammatory)
Key Vitamins & Minerals: Niacin (15% of RDA); B6 (14% of RDA) Thiamin (12% of RDA); Manganese (88% of RDA); Magnesium (21% of RDA).

Rye Bread
Serving: 1 slice
Calories: 83
Protein: 3 grams
Fiber: 2 grams
Carbohydrates: 15 grams
Fat: 1 gram
Sugars: 1 gram
Glycemic Load Index: 8
Inflammatory Rating: - 46 (mildly inflammatory)

Whole Wheat Bread
Serving: 1 slice
Calories: 69
Protein: 4 grams
Fiber: 2 grams
Carbohydrates: 12 grams
Fat: 1 gram
Sugars: 2 grams
Glycemic Load Index: 5
Inflammatory Rating: -28 (mildly inflammatory)
Key Vitamins & Minerals: Thiamin (7% of RDA); Manganese (30% of RDA); Selenium (16% of RDA).

Whole Wheat Pasta
Serving: 1 cup (cooked)
Calories: 174
Protein: 7 grams
Fiber: 6 grams
Carbohydrates: 37 grams
Fat: 1 gram
Sugars: 1 gram
Glycemic Load Index: 15
Inflammatory Rating: -81 (mildly inflammatory)
Key Vitamins & Minerals: Thiamin (10% of RDA); Manganese (97% of RDA); Selenium (52% of RDA).

Whole Wheat Cereal (unsweetened, dry, ready to eat) Serving: 1 cup (dry)
Calories: 213
Protein: 7 grams
Fiber: 6 grams
Carbohydrates: 44 grams
Fat: 2 grams
Sugars: 1 gram
Glycemic Load Index: 25
Inflammatory Rating: -184 (moderately inflammatory)
Key Vitamins & Minerals: A (15% of RDA); Iron 45% of RDA
Added milk: See Fertility Dairy for extra nutrients

Fertility Dairy

Cheese (Hard - Parmesan, cheddar, Swiss)
(Note: Counts may vary slightly by cheese type)
Serving: 1 ounce - full fat
Calories: 106
Protein: 8 grams
Fiber: 0
Carbohydrates: 2 grams
Fat: 8 grams (5 grams saturated)
Sugars: 0
Glycemic Load Index: 1
Inflammatory Rating: -24 (mildly inflammatory)
Key Vitamins & Minerals: Calcium (22% of RDA); B12 (16% of RDA)
A (5% of RDA) D (3% of RDA).

Cheese (Soft– Babybel, Brie, Feta, Mozzarella)
(Note: Counts may vary slightly by cheese type.)
Serving: 1 ounce
Calories: 94
Protein: 6 grams
Fiber: 0
Carbohydrates: 0
Fat: 8 grams (5 grams saturated)
Sugars: 0
Glycemic Load Index: 0
Inflammatory Rating: - 17 (mildly inflammatory)
Key Vitamins & Minerals: Selenium (6% of RDA); Calcium (5% of
RDA); Riboflavin (9% of RDA); B12 (8% of RDA) A (3% of RDA)

Cottage Cheese (Low Fat)
Serving: ½ cup
Calories: 81
Protein: 14 grams
Fiber: 0
Carbohydrates: 3 grams
Fat: 1 gram (saturated)
Sugars: 3 grams
Glycemic Load Index: 3
Inflammatory Rating: -14 (mildly inflammatory)
Key Vitamins & Minerals: Calcium (7% of RDA); Selenium (15% of RDA); B12 (12% of RDA) Riboflavin (11% of RDA).

Ice Cream (Breyers All Natural Vanilla - Light)
Serving: ½ cup
Calories: 110
Protein: 3 grams
Fiber: 0
Carbohydrates: 1 grams
Fat: 3 grams
Sugars: 15 grams
Glycemic Load Index: 9
Inflammatory Rating: n/a
Key Vitamins & Minerals: Calcium (11% of RDA) A (6% of RDA)

Ice Cream (Breyer's Vanilla - Full Fat)
Serving: ½ cup
Calories: 137
Protein: 2 grams
Fiber: 0
Carbohydrates: 16 grams
Fat: 7 grams (4 grams saturated)
Sugars: 14 grams
Glycemic Load Index: 8
Inflammatory Rating: -78 (mildly inflammatory)
Key Vitamins & Minerals : Calcium (8% of RDA); Riboflavin (9% of RDA) A (6% of RDA).

Cream Cheese (Regular)
Serving: 1 ounce
Calories: 96
Protein: 2 grams
Fiber: 0
Carbohydrates: 1 gram
Fat: 10 grams (5 grams saturated)
Sugars: 1 gram
Glycemic Load Index:0
Inflammatory Rating:- 48 (mildly inflammatory)
Key Vitamins & Minerals: A (7% of RDA) Calcium (3% of RDA)

Cream Cheese (Low Fat)
Serving: 1 ounce
Calories: 29
Protein: 4 grams
Fiber: 0
Carbohydrates: 2 grams
Fat: 0
Sugars: 2 grams
Glycemic Load Index: 1
Inflammatory Rating: - 6 (mildly inflammatory)
Key Vitamins & Minerals: Calcium (10% of RDA);
Phosphorus (15% of RDA) Riboflavin (4% of RDA)
B12 (4% of RDA)

Cottage Cheese (Regular)
Serving: ½ cup - regular
Calories: 111
Protein: 13 grams
Fiber: 0
Carbohydrates: 4 grams
Fat: 5 grams (2 gram saturated fat)
Sugars: 3 grams
Glycemic Load Index: 4
Inflammatory Rating: - 25 (mildly inflammatory)
Key Vitamins & Minerals: Calcium (9% of RDA); Selenium
(16% of RDA); Riboflavin (11% of RDA); B12 (8% RDA)

Milk (Whole)
Serving: 1 cup
Calories: 146
Protein: 8 grams
Fiber: 0
Carbohydrates: 13 grams
Fat: 8 grams (5 grams saturated fat)
Sugars: 13 grams
Glycemic Load Index: 9
Inflammatory Rating: - 77 (mildly inflammatory)
Key Vitamins & Minerals: Calcium (28% of RDA);
Phosphorus (22% of RDA); Vitamin D (24% of RDA)
Riboflavin (26% of RDA

Milk (Fat free or skim)
Serving: 1 cup
Calories: 83
Protein: 8 grams
Fiber: 0
Carbohydrates: 12 grams
Fat: 0
Sugars: 12 grams
Glycemic Load Index: 9
Inflammatory Rating: - 52 (mildly inflammatory)
Key Vitamins & Minerals: Calcium (31% of RDA)
(Note: Most brands are also fortified with Vitamin D; see the
label for the exact amount.

Yogurt (Regular)
Serving: 1 cup -unsweetened, plain
Calories: 149
Protein: 9 grams
Fiber: 0 (some brands are now fortified with fiber - check the label)
Carbohydrates: 11 grams
Fat: 8 grams (5 grams saturated)
Sugars: 11 grams
Glycemic Load Index: 9
Inflammatory Rating: -73 (mildly inflammatory)
Key Vitamins & Minerals: Calcium (30% of RDA); Riboflavin (20% of
RDA ; B12 (15% of RDA)

Yogurt (Low Fat)
Serving: 1 cup - unsweetened, plain
Calories: 154
Protein: 13 grams
Fiber: 0
Carbohydrates: 17 grams
Fat: 4 grams (2 grams saturated - can vary by brand)
Sugars: 17 grams (can vary by brand)
Glycemic Load Index: 10
Inflammatory Rating:- 71 (mildly inflammatory
Key Vitamins & Minerals: Calcium (45% of RDA);
Phosphorus (35% of RDA) ; Potassium (16% of RDA)
Riboflavin (31% of RDA); B12 (23% of RDA)

Yogurt (1% milkfat with strawberries)
Serving: 1 cup - sweetened
Calories: 218
Protein: 9 grams
Fiber: 0
Carbohydrates: 41 grams
Fat: 2 grams (1 gram saturated)
Sugars: 39 grams
Glycemic Load Index: 21
Inflammatory Rating: N/A
Key Vitamins & Minerals: Calcium (28% of RDA);
Phosphorus (20% of RDA); Potassium (12% of RDA);
Riboflavin (25% of RDA); B12 (12% of RDA)

If you don't like the taste of unsweetened yogurt, then buy the plain variety and add in your own fruit or even a spoonful of jam or preserves. You'll get the sweet taste with a much reduced level of sugar than what you'll find in pre-sweetened varieties!

Fertility Nuts & Seeds

Cashews
Serving: 1 ounce
Calories: 161
Protein: 4 grams
Fiber: 1 gram
Carbohydrates: 9 grams
Fat: 13 grams (3 grams saturated)
Sugars: 1 gram
Glycemic Load Index: 3
Inflammatory Rating: 22 (mildly anti-inflammatory
Key Vitamins & Minerals: K (12% of RDA); Copper (31% of RDA); Iron (9 % of RDA).

Flax Seeds
Serving: 1 ounce
Calories: 150
Protein: 5 grams
Fiber: 8 grams
Carbohydrates: 8 grams
Fat: 12 grams (1 gram saturated fat)
Sugars: 0
Glycemic Load Index: 0
Inflammatory Rating: 137 (mildly anti-inflammatory)
Key Vitamins & Minerals: Thiamin (31% of RDA); B6 (7 % of RDA)Manganese (35% of RDA); Magnesium (27% of RDA
BONUS: Omega 3 : 6,388 mg; Omega 6 : 1, 655 mg

Remember ... Nuts are good for fertility, but they are high in calories. So, eat them in moderation- you only need a handful thee times a week to get all the fertility-boosting benefits!

Peanuts (Dry Roasted)
Serving: 1 ounce
Calories: 164
Protein: 7 grams
Fiber: 2 grams
Carbohydrates: 6 grams
Fat: 14 grams (2 grams saturated fat)
Sugars: 1 gram
Glycemic Load Index: 0
Inflammatory Rating: 19 (mildly inflammatory)
Key Vitamins & Minerals: Manganese (29% of RDA); E (10% of RDA); Niacin (19% of RDA); Folate

Pumpkin Seeds
Serving: 1 ounce
Calories: 146
Protein: 9 grams
Fiber: 1 gram
Carbohydrates: 4 grams
Fat: 12 grams (2 grams saturated fat)
Sugars: 0
Glycemic Load Index: 0
Inflammatory Rating: - 24 (mildly inflammatory)
Key Vitamins & Minerals: Manganese (42% of RDA); Magnesium (37% of RDA); Phosphorus (33% of RDA); Iron (23% of RDA)

You can easily add seeds to your diet by crushing them in a food processor and then adding a handful to a cookie recipe, stews, even sauces. You won't taste the difference and you will boost the fertility power of every recipe!

Sunflower seeds (Dry Roasted)
Serving: 1 ounce
Calories: 163
Protein: 5 grams
Fiber: 3 grams
Carbohydrates: 7 grams
Fat: 14 grams (1 gram saturated)
Sugars: 1 gram
Glycemic Load Index: 0
Inflammatory Rating: - 40 (mildly

Key Vitamins & Minerals: E (37% of RDA) Selenium (32% of RDA)
Manganese (30% of RDA) Copper (26% of RDA)

Walnuts
Serving Size - 1 ounce (14 halves)
Calories : 185
Protein: 4 grams
Fiber: 2 grams
Carbohydrates : 4 grams
Fat : 18 grams (2 grams saturated
Sugars : 1 gram
Glycemic Load Index : 0
Inflammatory Rating - 38 (mildly inflammatory)
Key Vitamins & Minerals : Manganese (48% of R
Copper (22 % of RDA); B6 (8% of RDA
BONUS: Omega 3 - 2, 565 mg; Omega 6 - 10, 761 mg

Super Fertility Snack

Create a snack mix designed to boost fertility by combining a
handful of mini bite shredded wheat, some chopped nuts, a
handful of dried cranberries or blueberries and some
sunflower or pumpkin seeds. To add a bit of flavor, break
up a few whole wheat crackers
flavored with onion and garlic!

Healthy Fertility Fats & Oils

Canola Oil
Serving: 1 ounce
Calories: 248
Fat: 28 grams (2 grams saturated)
Glycemic Load Index: 0
Inflammatory Rating: 159 (moderately anti-inflammatory
Key Vitamins & Minerals: E (24% of RDA); K (25% of RDA)
Bonus: Omega 3 - 2, 559 mg ; Omega 6 - 5, 221 mg

Corn Oil
Serving: 1 ounce
Calories: 248
Fat: 28 grams (4 grams saturated)
Glycemic Load Index: 0
Inflammatory Rating: - 102 (mildly inflammatory)
Key Vitamins & Minerals: E (20% of RDA);
BONUS: Omega 3 - 325 mg ; Omega 6 - 14, 983

Grapeseed Oil
Serving: 1 ounce
Calories: 248
Fat: 28 grams (3 grams saturated)
Glycemic Load Index: 0
Inflammatory Rating: - 173 (moderately inflammatory)
Key Vitamins & Minerals: E (40% of RDA)
BONUS: Omega 3 - 28 mg; Omega 6 - 19, 485 mg

Olive Oil
Serving: 1 ounce
Calories:
Fats: 28 grams (4 grams saturated)
Glycemic Load Index : 0
Inflammatory Rating: 147 (moderately anti-inflammatory)
Key Vitamins & Minerals: E (20% of RDA); K (21% of RDA);
BONUS: Omega 3 - 213 mg; Omega 6: 2, 734

Safflower Oil
Serving: 1 ounce
Calories: 248
Fat: 28 grams (2 grams saturated)
Glycemic Load Index: 0
Inflammatory Rating: - 182 (moderately
Key Vitamins & Minerals: E (48% of RDA);
Bonus: Omega 6 - 20, 892 mg

Walnut Oil
Serving Size - 1 ounce
Calories : 248
Fat : 28 grams (3 grams saturated
Glycemic Load Index : 0
Inflammatory Rating - 51 (mildly inflammatory)
Key Vitamins & Minerals : K (5% of RDA)
BONUS: Omega 3 - 2, 912 mg ; Omega 6 - 14, 810 mg

Mayonaise (Regular)
Serving Size: 1 tablespoon
Calories: 109
Fat: 12 grams (2 grams saturated - this can vary by brands)
Glycemic Load Index : 0
Inflammatory Rating - 33 (mildly inflammatory)
Key Vitamins & Minerals: E (9% of RDA);
Bonus: Omega 3 - 745 mg; Omega 5 - 6, 085 mg

Mayonnaise (low fat)
Serving: 1 tablespoon
Calories: 48
Fat: 5 grams (1 gram saturated - this can vary by brands)
Glycemic Load Index: 0
Inflammatory Rating - 14 (mildly inflammatory)
Key Vitamins & Minerals: E (5% of RDA)
Bonus: Omega 3 - 309 mg; Omega 6 - 519 mg

Fertility Meat & Poultry

Chicken - Roasted
Serving: ½ breast - skin and bone removed
Calories: 142
Protein: 27 grams
Fiber: 0
Carbohydrates: 0
Fat: 3 grams (1 gram saturated)
Sugars: 0
Glycemic Load Index: 0
Inflammatory Rating: - 18 (mildly inflammatory)
Key Vitamins & Minerals: Niacin (59% of RDA) B6 (26% RDA)
Selenium (34% RDA);
Bonus: Omega 3 - 60.2 mg; Omega 6 - 507 mg

Turkey (Roasted)
Scrving: 3.5 oz white meat
Calories : 135
Protein: 30 grams
Fiber: 0
Carbohydrates: 0
Fat: 1 gram
Sugars: 0
Glycemic Load Index: 0
Inflammatory Rating - 3 (mildly inflammatory)
Key Vitamins & Minerals: Niacin (37% of RDA) B6 (28% of RDA)
Bonus: Omega 3 - 20 mg; Omega 6: 130 mg

Beef (Ground - 95% lean)
Serving: 3.5 oz - broiled
Calories: 171
Protein: 26 grams
Fiber: 0
Carbohydrates : 0
Fat: 7 grams (3 grams saturated fat)
Sugars: 0
Glycemic Load Index: 0
Inflammatory Rating: -12 (mildly inflammatory)
Key Vitamins & Minerals: B12 (41% of RDA); Niacin (30% of RDA); Zinc (43% of RDA); Selenium (31% of RDA)

Beef (Roasted, trimmed to 0 visible fat)
Serving:3.5 oz -roasted
Calories: 211
Protein: 26 grams
Fiber: 0
Carbohydrates: 0
Fats: 11 grams (4 grams saturated fat)
Sugars: 0
Glycemic Load Index: 0
Inflammatory Rating: 16 (mildly anti-inflammatory)
Key Vitamins & Minerals: Niacin (9% of RDA) B6 (8% of RDA) B12 (5 % of RDA) Iron (2 % of RDA.

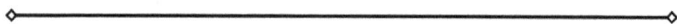

◇———————————————————◇

If there a difference between 85% & 90% lean ground beef? You bet there is! This simple 5% reduction in fat can not only save a ton of calories but also reduce the inflammatory factors & the saturated fat! And that can be very good for fertility!

Fertility Fish

Cod Filet
Serving: 3 ounces
Calories: 105
Protein: 23 grams
Fiber: 0
Carbohydrates: 0
Fat: 1 gram
Sugars: 0
Glycemic Load Index: 0
Inflammatory Rating: 81 (mildly anti-inflammatory)
Key Vitamins & Minerals: B12 (18% of RDA); B6 (14% of RDA); Selenium (54% of RDA;
BONUS: Omega 3 - 172 mg; Omega 6 -6 mg

Flatfish (Flounder or Sole)
Serving: 3 ounces
Calories: 99
Protein: 21 grams
Fiber: 0
Carbohydrates: 0
Fats:1 gram
Sugars:
Glycemic Load Index: 0
Inflammatory Rating - 202 (moderately anti-inflammatory)
Key Vitamins & Minerals: B12 (36% of RDA); B6 (10% of RDA); Selenium (71% of RDA);
Bonus: Omega 3- 478 mg; Omega 6 - 11.9 mg

Salmon (Canned)
Serving: 3.5 ounces (drained, with bones)
Calories: 136
Protein: 23 grams
Fiber: 0
Carbohydrates: 1 gram
Fat: 5 (1 gram saturated fat)
Sugars: 0
Glycemic Load Index: 0
Inflammatory Rating: 500 (strongly anti-inflammatory)
Key Vitamins & Minerals: D (117% of RDA); B12 (82% of
RDA); Niacin (37% of RDA); Calcium (28% of RDA);
Selenium (56% of RDA); Phosphorus (36% of RDA)
Bonus: Omega 3 - 1,210 mg; Omega 6- 95 mg

Salmon (Fresh, wild)
Serving: 5.3 ounces
Calories: 280
Protein: 39 grams
Fiber: 0
Carbohydrates: 0
Fats: 13 grams (2 grams saturated)
Sugars:0
Glycemic Load Index: 0
Inflammatory Rating: 895 (strongly anti-inflammatory)
Key Vitamins & Minerals: B12 (73% of RDA); Niacin (78%
of RDA); Copper (25% of RDA);
Bonus: Omega 3 - 3,982 mg; Omega 6 - 339 mg

One of the most nutritious "fertility foods" you can eat is fish! The Omega 3 fatty acids offer amazing fertility benefits and they can be especially helpful if you suffer with endometriosis or PCOS!

Sardines (canned, in tomato sauce)
Serving: 3.5 ounces
Calories: 186 grams
Protein: 21 grams
Fiber: 0
Carbohydrates: 1 gram
Fat: 10 grams (3 grams saturated fat)
Sugars: 0
Glycemic Load Index: 1
Inflammatory Rating: 422 (strongly anti-inflammatory)
Key Vitamins & Minerals: B12 (150% of RDA); D (120% of RDA); Niacin (21% of RDA); Selenium (58% of RDA)
Bonus: Omega 3 - 1, 693 mg; Omega 6 - 123 mg

Shrimp (boiled or grilled)
Serving: 3.5 ounces
Calories : 99
Protein: 21 grams
Fiber: 0
Carbohydrates: 0
Fats: 1 gram Sugars:
Glycemic Load Index: 0
Inflammatory Rating : 115 (mildly anti-inflammatory) Key Vitamins & Minerals: B12 (25% of RDA); Niacin (13% of RDA); Selenium (57% of RDA)
Bonus: Omega 3 - 347 mg; Omega 6 - 21 mg

Shrimp (Batter Dipped/ Fried)
Serving: 3 oz.
Calories: 206
Protein: 18 grams
Fiber: 0
Carbohydrates: 10 grams
Fats: 10 grams (2 grams saturated)
Sugars: 0
Glycemic Load Index: 5
Inflammatory Rating: 25 (mildly anti-inflammatory)
Key Vitamins & Minerals: B12 (26% of RDA); Niacin (13% of RDA); Selenium (51% of RDA); Copper (12% of RDA)
Bonus: Omega 3 - 455 mg; Omega 6: 3, 834 mg

Tuna (White - canned)
Serving: 1 can (6 ounces)
Calories: 220
Protein: 41 grams
Fiber: 0
Carbohydrates: 0
Fats: 5 grams (1 gram saturated)
Sugars: 0
Glycemic Load Index: 0
Inflammatory Rating: 698 (strongly anti-inflammatory)
Key Vitamins & Minerals: Niacin (50% of RDA); B12 (34% of RDA); Selenium (161 % of RDA);
Bonus: Omega 3 - 1, 636 mg; Omega 6 - 94.6 mg

Tuna (Fresh - Bluefin)
Serving: 3 ounces raw (sushi)
Calories: 122
Protein: 20 grams
Fiber: 0
Carbohydrates: 0
Fats: 4 grams (1 gram saturated fat)
Sugars: 0
Glycemic Load Index: 0
Inflammatory Rating: 464 (strongly anti-inflammatory)
Key Vitamins & Minerals: A (37% RDA) ; Niacin (37% of RDA); Selenium (44% of RDA);
Bonus: Omega 3 - 1, 103 mg; Omega 6 - 45 mg.

◇————————————————◇

*If you purchase canned tuna, always chose white meat only -
and do check the labels among different brands.
Many contain preservatives you might want to avoid. When
possible seek out all - natural tuna packed in spring water only -
with no vegetable broth added.*

Fertility Height & Weight Chart

To optimize your fertility, use the following
chart to determine whether you need to
lose or gain weight.

If your Height is:	Your Best Fertility Weight is:
4'10"	109 - 121
4'11"	111 - 123
5'0"	113- 126
5'1"	115 - 129
5'2"	118 -132
5'3"	121- 135
5'4"	124 -138
5'5"	127-141
5'6"	130-144
5'7"	133-147
5'8"	136-150
5'9"	139-153
5'10"	142-156
5'11"	145-159
6'0"	148-162

Note: Height includes 1" heels; weight includes 3 pounds of clothes.

Important Note:

When figuring your proper fertility weight you must also take into consideration your body type and bone structure.

To do so use the following formula:

Small Bones:
   Wrist Measurement: 5.5" or less
   Ankle Measurement: 8" or less

Large bones:
   Wrist Measurement: 6" or more.
   Ankle Measurement: 9" or more

For small bones use the number on the lower end of the weight chart; for large bones, use the higher number.

Body Mass Index

Body Mass Index or BMI is a way of using your height and weight to calculate your level of body fat.

While a BMI calculation does not measure your body fat directly, the results do correlate with tests that do - such as underwater weighing, or a type of special x-ray known as absorptiometry (DXA).

Since, however, both these tests can be expensive - and the BMI is free for anyone to use - it's easy to see why it's become one of the most popular ways to determine levels of body fat.

As a fertility doctor I have also found the BMI helpful in identifying women at risk for some specific weight -related fertility problems. Indeed, when a woman's BMI is too low (indicating she has too little body fat) or too high (indicating she has too much body fat) it can impact her ability to get pregnant.

To find your BMI and further determine your fertility weight status, use the chart on the next page.

BMI - Body Mass Index Chart

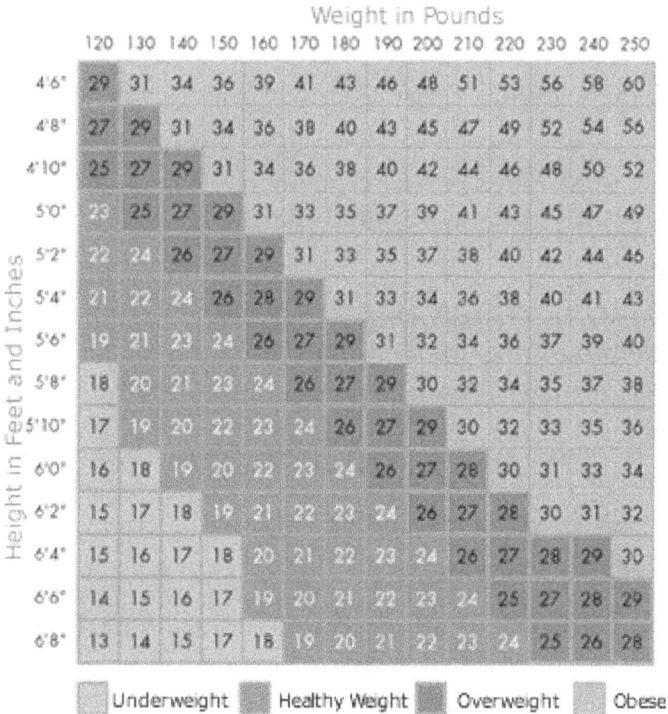

Weight in Pounds

Height	120	130	140	150	160	170	180	190	200	210	220	230	240	250
4'6"	29	31	34	36	39	41	43	46	48	51	53	56	58	60
4'8"	27	29	31	34	36	38	40	43	45	47	49	52	54	56
4'10"	25	27	29	31	34	36	38	40	42	44	46	48	50	52
5'0"	23	25	27	29	31	33	35	37	39	41	43	45	47	49
5'2"	22	24	26	27	29	31	33	35	37	38	40	42	44	46
5'4"	21	22	24	26	28	29	31	33	34	36	38	40	41	43
5'6"	19	21	23	24	26	27	29	31	32	34	36	37	39	40
5'8"	18	20	21	23	24	26	27	29	30	32	34	35	37	38
5'10"	17	19	20	22	23	24	26	27	29	30	32	33	35	36
6'0"	16	18	19	20	22	23	24	26	27	28	30	31	33	34
6'2"	15	17	18	19	21	22	23	24	26	27	28	30	31	32
6'4"	15	16	17	18	20	21	22	23	24	26	27	28	29	30
6'6"	14	15	16	17	19	20	21	22	23	24	25	27	28	29
6'8"	13	14	15	17	18	19	20	21	22	23	24	25	26	28

Height in Feet and Inches

Underweight   Healthy Weight   Overweight   Obese

Instructions: Find your height (in inches) in the column to the left; find your weight in pounds across the top; where the two numbers meet is your approximate BMI.

Example: If your height is 64" (5'4") and your weight is 143 pounds, your BMI would be approximately 26.

Once you know your BMI, go to the next chart on the next page to determine your fertility risk evaluation.

Know Your Fertility Weight Risks!

Now that you have your BMI it's time to use that information to access your weight-related fertility risks. To make that easier, all BMI results fall into one of six categories: Underweight, Normal Weight, Overweight, Obese 1, Obese 2 and Extremely Obese.

So the first step in determining your risks is to use the chart on the following page to determine in which of these categories your BMI measurement falls. Because, however, it's not just your level of body fat that is important, but where that fat is concentrated - the next step requires that you take one more measurement. Indeed, as you read earlier, body fat that is located in the belly region is particularly harmful to fertility - so that is the measurement you need to determine right now.

To do this I'm going to ask you to grab a tape measure and determine if your waist is less than, equal to or greater than 35 inches. (For men, by the way, the key number is 40 inches).

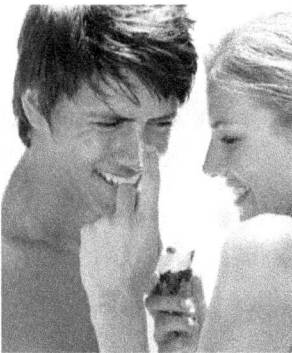

The latest research shows that being overweight can also impact male fertility, reducing sperm production and making it harder to fertilize an egg! So, make sure your partner follows these BMI guidelines too!

Fertility Risk Assessment Chart

Risk of Weight Related Fertility Problems

BMI	Weight Category	Waist: 35" or less	Waist: 36" Plus
18.5 or less	Underweight	Increased	_____
18.5 - 24.9	Normal	_____	_____
25.0 - 29.9	Overweight	Increased	High
30.0 -34.9	Obese	High	Very High
35.0 - 39.9	Obese	Very High	Very High
40 or greater	Extremely Obese	Extremely High	Extremely High

To Determine Your Fertility Risks:

Using the chart above find your BMI in the column on the left. Then follow across that line to determine your level of risk.

Example: If your BMI is 26 and your waist is 33" your risk of a fertility problem is "Increased". If your waist is 37" then your risk of fertility related problem is "high"

Definition of Probability Odds:

INCREASED RISK: 50% or more likely to have a problem getting pregnant.
HIGH RISK: 50-70% likely to have a problem conceiving.
VERY HIGH RISK: 80% likely to have a problem conceiving.
EXTREMELY HIGH RISK : 90- 98% likely to have a problem getting pregnant.

THE GOOD NEWS: By watching your diet and normalizing your weight you can completely turn your fertility odds around and get pregnant fast! Check my 7 Day Caloric Guide on the following page for help in reaching your goals.

7 Day Calorie Counting Guide

To help you determine the correct number of calories necessary to lose, gain or maintain the proper fertility weight, use the following calorie guide.

If you are 5'4" or under you should aim for the lower number in the calorie range; if you are 5'5" or taller, use the higher number as your target goal.

If you want to lose weight: Your daily caloric intake should be between 1400 and 1800 calories or between 9,800 and 12,600 per week - divided in any way you choose.

If you want to gain weight: Your daily caloric intake should be between 2100 and 2400 calories daily or between 14,700 and 16,800 calories per week, divided any way you like.

If you want to maintain your weight: Continue eating in your normal fashion. For most women of normal weight caloric intake is about 2,000 to 2,200 calories daily, or between 14,000 and 15,4 00 calories per week.

IMPORTANT NOTE: These calorie counts are to be used in conjunction with a moderate exercise program that includes at least 30 minutes of exercise 4 to 5 days per week.

Disclaimer: Every woman's body type if different - and every woman's metabolism is unique. For this reason the caloric intake suggestions in this section are just that - suggestions. To achieve your personal fertility weight goals your caloric intake may have to deviate from this guide. It's important that you check with your doctor before starting any weight loss program and be mindful of his or her opinion and suggestions concerning your weight and your fertility.

About
Niels H. Lauersen, M.D., Ph.D

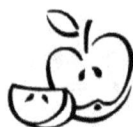

Born in Copenhagen, Denmark and educated throughout the capitols of Europe as an obsetrician/gynecologist and fertility expert, Dr. Niels Lauersen has dedicated more than 30 years to treating and educating women about their health in both the US and abroad.

He is the author of over 100 medical papers published in top journals worldwide and he is the author of 8 books on women's health, including his now-classic best sellers "It's Your Body" and the international best selling **"Getting Pregnant: What You Need To Know Now.**

Dr. Lauersen is also the medical director of the fertility website www.GettingPregnantNow.org

Contact him directly at: DrLauersen@Gmail.com

About
Colette Bouchez

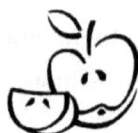

Colette Bouchez is an award-winning medical journalist and former content producer of women's health at WebMD. She is the author of 8 books on women's health and wellness including, Your Perfectly Pampered Pregnancy, The V Zone: A Woman's Guide To Intimate Health, and with Dr. Lauersen, **"Getting Pregnant: What You Need To Know Now."**

Colette's online syndicated column, **RedDressDiary.com** is seen weekly by over 2 million women and regularly appears in such newspapers as The Detroit Free Press, The Burlington Free Press, The Chicago Sun Times, USA Today and many others.

Contact Colette at : Colette Bouchez@aol.com or visit her website at www.ColetteBouchez.com

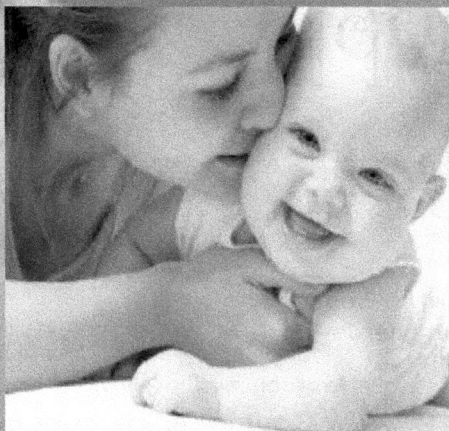

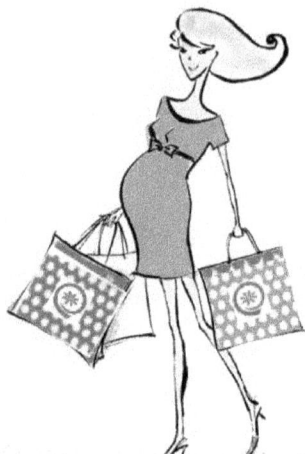

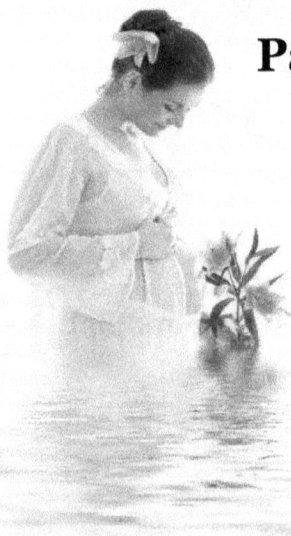

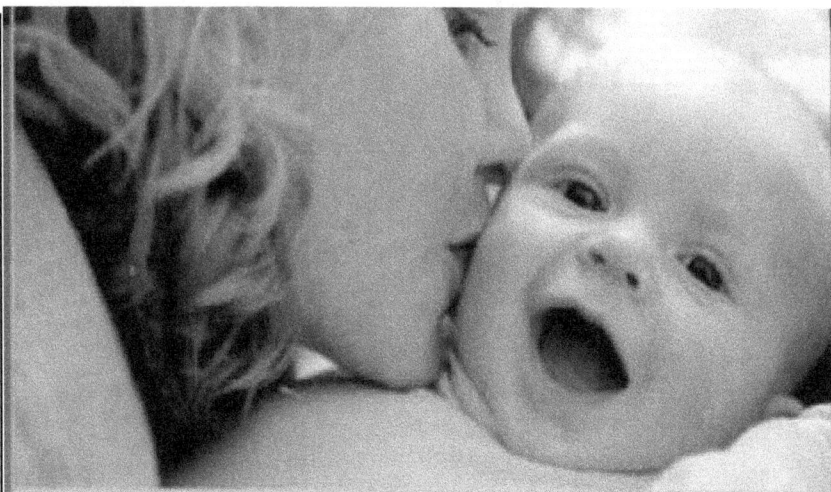

The Classic Best Seller - Completely Revised and Updated

Getting Pregnant

WHAT YOU NEED TO KNOW RIGHT NOW

BREAKTHROUGH TECHNIQUES FOR
TREATING INFERTILITY PLUS;

How to get pregnant fast -
Six new ways to avoid miscarriage
Pre Conception Exam -
The vitamins, minerals
& herbs that encourage fertility .
How To choose the sex of your baby -
And much more!

By Niels H. Lauersen, MD, PhD & Colette Bouchez

Getting Pregnant:
What You Need To Know Now!

From the authors of **The New Fertility Diet Guide** comes the top selling book on getting pregnant for nearly two decades! Now fully updated, discover why tens of thousands of couples already call this book their "Fertility Bible".

Voted # 1 by New Moms Worldwide this is the quintessential guide to everything you need to get pregnant fast!

A small fraction of what you'll find inside:

** The fastest, easiest ways to a safe, natural conception.

** What to do today to double your chance for conception tomorrow!

** All Natural Male Fertility Boosters!
** Getting Pregnant after a vasectomy.
** Six new ways to prevent miscarriage
** How to get pregnant naturally - after age 40!

Plus:

- **8 brand new fertility drugs - including which ones are the safest .**
- **The new 15 minute in-office surgery that can double conception odds immediately!**
- **The latest versions of IVF , GIFT and IUI.**
- **The hottest new medical treatments**
- **AND SO MUCH MORE!**

Visit www.GetPregnantFast.net to discover how to purchase this amazing book in print - or as an Ebook! At fine bookstores nationwide and online !

www.ingramcontent.com/pod-product-compliance
Lightning Source LLC
Chambersburg PA
CBHW050121280326
41933CB00010B/1189